OXFORD MEDICAL PUE

P9-CKR-818

MULTIPLE
SCLEROSIS

LEGE

DATE DUE

the**facts**

ALSO AVAILABLE IN THE SERIES

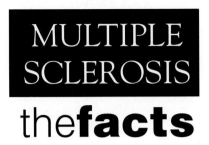

MULTIPLE SCLEROSIS

the**facts**

Fourth Edition

Bryan Matthews DM FRCP
Emeritus Professor of Clinical Neurology
University of Oxford

and

Margaret Rice-Oxley
Consultant in Rehabilitation Medicine
St. Richard's Hospital
Chichester
West Sussex

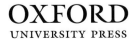

OXFORD
UNIVERSITY PRESS

OXFORD
UNIVERSITY PRESS

Great Clarendon Street, Oxford OX2 6DP

Oxford University Press is a department of the University of Oxford.
It furthers the University's objective of excellence in research,
scholarship,and education by publishing worldwide in

Oxford   New York

Athens   Auckland   Bangkok   Bogotá   Buenos Aires   Cape Town
Chennai   Dar es Salaam   Delhi   Florence   Hong Kong   Istanbul
Karachi   Kolkata   Kuala Lumpur   Madrid   Melbourne
Mexico City   Mumbai   Nairobi   Paris   São Paulo   Singapore
Taipei   Tokyo   Toronto   Warsaw

and associated companies in Berlin   Ibadan

Oxford is a registered trade mark of Oxford University Press
in the UK and in certain other countries

Published in the United States
by Oxford University Press Inc., New York

First edition published 1978
First edition published as an Oxford University Press paperback with
revisions 1980
Second edition 1985
Third edition 1993
Fourth edition 2001

British Library Cataloguing in Publication Data

Data available

Library of Congress Cataloguing in Publication Data

ISBN 0 19 850898 0

10 9 8 7 6 5 4 3 2 1

Typeset by Expo Holdings Sdn Bhd
Printed in Great Britain
on acid-free paper by

Biddles Ltd, Guildford & King's Lynn

Professor Bryan Matthews died peacefully shortly before publication of this, his last book.

Although I helped him with it, I insisted that he rewrote my chapter on 'Coping with MS' in his own style in order to maintain his wonderfully personal way of writing. All the neurologists who have worked with him will be able to 'hear' him talking to his patients throughout these chapters. He always felt real pain in imparting the diagnosis of multiple sclerosis, but he never patronised people, and many people with MS greatly appreciated his clear and frank approach in previous editions of this book.

All of us who worked with Bryan will mourn the loss of a loyal and witty friend.

Margaret Rice-Oxley

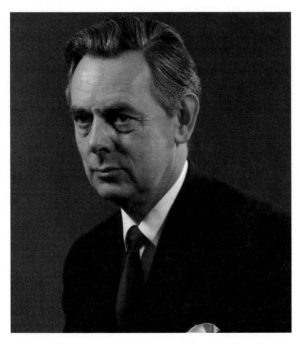

Professor Bryan Matthews b. 7 April 1920; d. 12 July 2001.

Preface to the fourth edition

Earlier editions of this book were written by a single author (BM) but it clearly became essential to expand the detailed account of the day-to-day care of people with MS, particularly of those with more severe disabilities. This need has been met by an expert in rehabilitation (M R-O) with extensive and continuing experience of hands-on care. We decided not to become involved in distinctions of 'I' or 'we' and that the personal style of the book should as far as possible be retained.

the**facts**

CONTENTS

1
What is multiple sclerosis?

Although there had been earlier partial descriptions, multiple sclerosis was first identified as a distinctive disease in 1868 by the great French neurologist Charcot, working at the Salpêtrière hospital in Paris. It is strange that a disease that now seems to be so well defined should have remained unrecognized for so long, but methods of examining someone with organic disease of the nervous system were only then being developed. Charcot's great contribution to medicine was in linking the careful observation of symptoms and signs of disease in life with the pathological findings in the nervous system after death. He called this new disease '*sclérose en plaques*' a phrase that in his original lecture he feared would sound barbarous to his audience. The 'sclérose' or sclerosis of his title means hardening and refers to the scarring that is the end result of the damage caused to the nervous system by multiple sclerosis. The word 'sclerosis' was used very freely in the early days of neurology and persists in the confusing title used in the United States to describe a quite different and much more serious disease of the nervous system, amyotrophic lateral sclerosis (ALS).

The word is used elsewhere in medicine, for example in arteriosclerosis, or hardening of the arteries, that has nothing to do with multiple sclerosis. Another source of confusion is with the word 'cirrhosis' usually applied to the liver and originally referring to the yellow colour sometimes displayed by that organ when diseased. This again has no connection with multiple sclerosis.

The word 'plaque', still very much in use in the study of multiple sclerosis, literally means a tablet, that is, something with a flat surface. This is a misconception of the nature of the individual areas of damage to the nervous system—the lesions—and is derived from the appearance of such a lesion cut across and viewed with the naked eye or through a microscope. As can be seen from Figure 1 this naturally presents a flat surface—the plaque—but this is merely a cross-section of a lesion that may extend a considerable distance through the nervous system. In Great Britain the disease was originally known as disseminated sclerosis, shortened to DS, a name that emphasized the feature of plaques scattered throughout the central nervous system. Gradually, this name was replaced by that popular in the United States— multiple sclerosis or MS. The main reason for the change was the existence of the Multiple Sclerosis Society of America and the importance attached to ensuring that the Society of Great Britain was similarly named. Disseminated and multiple sclerosis are the same disease.

The nervous system

To understand the impact of MS it is necessary to have some knowledge of the anatomy of the

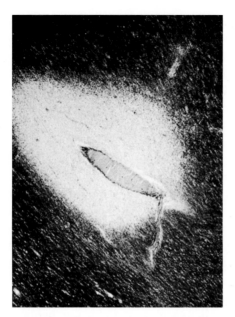

Figure 1. This is a section of a small plaque. The tissue has been stained so the myelin shows as black, and the sharp contrast between the white plaque and the surrounding normal brain tissue is striking. The magnification is not high enough to show individual nerve fibres. In the centre is a small vein that has been cut across obliquely.

nervous system and of how it works. The central nervous system (CNS) consists of the brain, within the skull, and the spinal cord running down the centre of the backbone. These are not, of course, separate organs but join at the base of the skull. The CNS communicates with the muscles and receives information from sensory organs through the peripheral nervous system that branches throughout the body. This distinction between peripheral and central is important as the lesions of MS are strictly confined to the CNS. The optic nerves that connect the eyeballs to the brain are also part of the CNS and are frequently affected in MS, but apart from this the plaques occur in the brain and spinal cord only.

The CNS performs a great variety of functions, based on the receipt and analysis of information from the outside world and from internal organs, and the initiation and control of the response, whether this be movement, emotion, or some more basic activity, such as sweating or emptying the bladder. However, the nervous system does not act solely as an automatic machine, and there is much that is controversial or unknown, particularly with regard to functions such as consciousness, memory, and reason. All these functions depend on the nerve cells (or neurons) of which the brain contains many millions, linked in an orderly but inconceivably complex manner. Each neuron consists of a cell body and a variable number of elongated processes, of which the nerve fibre (axon) is of particular importance in MS. It is along the axon that the nervous impulse, generated in the cell body, passes on its way to link with other neurons in the CNS or, via the peripheral nervous system, to other organs such as muscles or secretory glands. The impulse, that involves both electrical and chemical changes, travels at different speeds according to the diameter of the axon seen in cross-section, conduction being faster in the largest fibres. To give an idea of scale, the diameter of the largest fibres is about one-fiftieth of a millimetre. The large fibres, and also many of smaller diameter, are surrounded by a sheath of a complex chemical containing protein and lipid, or fat, and is known as myelin. This is laid down in a discontinuous spiral manner around the length of the axon

(Figure 2) interrupted every millimetre or so by a short bare segment known as a node.

Myelin, although a chemical, is laid down and supported within a living cell. These cells are much

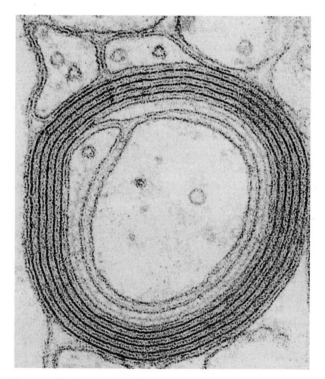

Figure 2. This shows the normal appearance of a nerve fibre or axon surrounded by spiral layers of myelin. This is shown in cross-section enormously magnified under an electron microscope. It is difficult to obtain such beautiful pictures except under experimental conditions and this is a myelinated fibre in a rat. Human fibres are similar, but in most there will be many more spiral layers. At the top of the figure is the oligodendrocyte responsible for laying down the myelin sheath.

easier to study in the peripheral nervous system and most experimental work has been done there. However, in the CNS it is a particular form of cell that is responsible for the myelin. The neuroglial, or glial, cells are the other main component of the CNS and are concerned with many supporting activities, such as the nutrition of neurons, and with the healing process. It is the group recognized under the formidable title of the oligodendrocytes (cells with few branches) that is responsible for forming the myelin sheath, each short segment between two nodes being formed and maintained by one oligo-dendrocyte. The functions of the myelin sheaths are not fully known. The comparison with an insulated electric wire, with the conducting axon in the centre surrounded by insulating myelin, is certainly too simple but myelin has an important role in accelerating conduction along the axon.

Plaques

Probably the first event in the formation of a plaque is that lymphocytes (a form of white blood cell) begin to adhere to the walls of small blood vessels in the CNS. These lymphocytes have been activated, presumably by contact with an antigen, as yet unknown, which is recognized as harmful, causing them to behave abnormally. They then penetrate the tight wall of cells lining the blood vessels, thus breaking the blood–brain barrier that normally affords some protection to the CNS from changes in the composition of the blood and also prevents the passage of white blood cells. The lymphocytes pen-etrate the tissue of the CNS and secrete substances (lymphokines) that cause inflammation, swelling with excess fluid, and antibodies to myelin and oligodendrocytes; all of these factors block or reduce conduction in axons. Failure to conduct will cause symptoms if the plaque is in a strategic site where axons are tightly packed, such as the optic nerve or spinal cord, but many plaques seen on MRI scans (see Chapter 5) cause no symptoms at all.

As time passes, the broken-down myelin is removed by scavenger cells and there is an increase in another form of neuroglial cells, the astrocytes, so called from their star-shaped appearance in stained sections under the microscope, and it is these cells that form the scarring or sclerosis. The lymphocytes disappear from the centre of the plaque but may persist at the edge where the disease process is still active (Figure 3). Many axons escape intact but even at this early stage some may be lost.

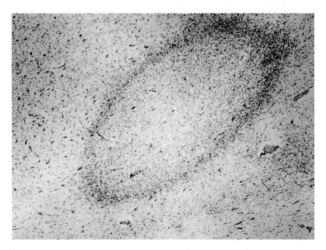

Figure 3. An MS plaque in the brain stained to show the lymphocytes as dark dots forming a ring. This intense activity indicates that the plaque was extending all around the periphery.

Spontaneous recovery from the early symptoms of MS is the rule but it is not obvious from examination of the plaques how this happens. Authoritative statements were made that in MS myelin could not be re-formed. This is surprising, as remyelination is common in diseases quite distinct from MS that cause extensive loss of myelin in the peripheral nervous system followed by recovery from severe paralysis. In some plaques the axons are surrounded by abnormally thin myelin sheaths. This had been interpreted as myelin in the course of destruction, but opinion has veered strongly towards regarding these 'shadow plaques' as areas of remyelination in progress. If this is so, it could be one factor in the recovery from symptoms in a remission. Unfortunately, at some stage, remyelination fails as by the time they are examined most plaques are devoid of myelin. Other factors that are certainly important both in the production of symptoms and in the initial rapid recovery are the swelling and inflammation in the plaques. The excess fluid can exert pressure on the bared axons and block conduction, which would be at least partially restored when the swelling subsided, even in the absence of myelin sheaths.

These then are the plaques. By the time the nervous system can be examined there are usually many plaques in different stages of development scattered throughout the CNS, thus referred to as 'multiple'. They are largely confined to the white matter that consists mostly of myelinated axons whereas in the grey matter neurons predominate (Figure 5, p. 53). As seen on MRI scans, plaques are often multiple from the onset even when the symptoms and signs suggest a single lesion. Even in advanced cases plaques do not seem to be scattered entirely at random. They are never completely symmetrical but show a strong tendency to develop on both sides at certain, apparently vulnerable, sites including the optic nerves and the spinal cord in the neck.

The pattern of MS

Despite extensive research and many false trails there is little to suggest that MS could be a generalized disease in the sense that tuberculosis, for example, can affect many different organs and systems of the body. MS does not directly affect the lungs, heart, skin, or kidneys. The only exception is the inflammation of small blood vessels in the retina and of part of the eye known as the uvea. Both of these conditions also occur for no known reason in people who do not have MS.

The relapsing and remitting course and other features of the pattern of disease in MS are not entirely unfamiliar, as there are obvious parallels with certain diseases of the skin. Here, too, there is often no sign of general ill health and the colloquial name 'spots' indicates that the disease is patchy, with most of the skin free from blemish. Certain forms of urticaria or nettle rash, and some rashes caused by sensitivity to drugs bear a close resemblance to some of the features of MS. Particular areas of skin are involved, seemingly at random, whereas the rest is spared, although the noxious agent must be present throughout the body. The rash comes and goes, often with long intervals of freedom, and returns, often without a recognizable reason. Particularly striking is the rash known as a fixed drug eruption.

Here, in response to a minute dose of a drug to which the patient's skin is sensitive or allergic, large round plaques of inflammation appear haphazardly on the body surface. These persist for a number of weeks, fading gradually, but if a second dose is taken they extend from the edges in a fresh ring. The capacity of the skin for healing exceeds that of the CNS and no permanent harm ensues even after repeated attacks so the comparison must not be pursued too far. However, this is another disease, at first sight quite mysterious, producing multiple disseminated plaques with intervals of recovery. Even in skin diseases where the course can so easily be followed the cause may be difficult to uncover, but when once found prevention can be completely successful.

There is, of course, no connection at all between skin eruptions and MS and the example is given simply to illustrate that the relapsing and remitting course so characteristic of the early stages of the disease is not unique. The onset takes this form in about 80% of people with MS. The subsequent course of MS is described in later chapters.

2 Who gets multiple sclerosis?

There are many unusual facts concerning the distribution of MS in the world population which must be taken into account in any comprehensive theory of cause of the disease. Before describing these I must emphasize that all figures relating to the prevalence of MS are approximate. Early cases are often not diagnosed because the symptoms have been slight or fleeting. The figures are also influenced in the opposite direction because, no matter how careful the examination, there are always some patients thought to have MS who are subsequently found to have some quite different disease. Investigators are forced to classify their patients in separate categories of diagnostic certainty or doubt, the most usual being: possible, probable, or definite, as defined by clinical features, now assisted by results of laboratory and imaging tests. The difficulties in diagnosis must be remembered when discussing the pattern of who gets MS and who does not.

Age of onset

MS is rare in childhood. I have personally observed only two children under the age of 10 with symptoms and signs characteristic of the disease in adults. An acute form may also occur in children but is difficult to distinguish from other causes of encephalitis (inflammation of the brain) and are unlikely to be of interest to anyone reading this book. The frequency of onset of MS begins to increase around the age of 17 and reaches a peak in the early 30s. Thereafter, the onset becomes increasingly uncommon, but new cases without any past history at all suggestive of earlier attacks, continue to occur into the 60s. Where notes are available, either from hospital or from the family doctor, it is astonishing how easily people forget symptoms sufficiently severe to lead them to seek medical advice or even leading to admission to hospital, so the age of onset of symptoms must again be an approximation. However, it is well known that the diagnosis may be made by finding a few scattered plaques at a routine post-mortem examination in people who died in their 80s without apparently ever having experienced symptoms that could be attributed to MS. It is young adults and the middle-aged who bear the brunt of the disease. In virtually every research series reported women are more frequently affected than men, the usual ratio being three women to two men.

Prevalence of MS

There are two common methods of expressing the prevalence with which a disease occurs in a given population. The annual incidence is the number of new cases recorded every year in some stated number, often per 100 000 of the population. The prevalence of a disease is the number of people, again in 100 000, known to have the disease on a given day. The former figure is obviously the one to use when dealing with acute short-lived diseases like influenza, whereas the prevalence rate is the more useful for most purposes in a chronic disease like MS. These figures are partly dependent on the standard of medical care, the number of doctors capable of distinguishing MS from other nervous diseases, and the accuracy with which the facts are collected and published. In many parts of the world figures are poor or non-existent. In many tropical countries, although no attempt at precision can be made, a fair idea of relative prevalence can be formed. Despite these deficiencies there is an impressive body of evidence from around the world for a striking pattern of distribution. The prevalence of MS varies markedly according to geography, and with some notable exceptions, the most obvious factor involved is distance from the equator.

Geographical location

In tropical countries, for which any estimate can be made, MS is rare or does not occur at all in the indigenous population. In India, occasional small series of people with MS have been reported, particularly among Parsees, but it is plain that general prevalence is low. In contrast, in north-west Europe and in the northern states of the United States and in Canada prevalence is high, that is, above 40 per 100 000. This is also true of southern Australia and New Zealand. In Great Britain, general prevalence is around 100 per 100 000 but even here the figure is higher in northern latitudes, and in the Orkneys prevalence reached over 300 per 100 000, the highest in the world in 1974, but most interestingly, has since fallen. If the effect on prevalence is entirely due to latitude the rate in Japan would be expected to resemble that in Great Britain, but MS is comparatively rare in Japan (although more severe). There are other anomalies showing that simple distance from the equator or some secondary effect of this, such as temperature, cannot be the only factor concerned; for example, MS is common in Sicily but rare in neighbouring Malta.

It is not easy to visualize the significance of such figures in everyday terms. One hundred per 100 000 is 2 per 2000, one person with MS in a large village, or in one doctor's practice. Put like that the prevalence scarcely sounds 'high', but it has been calculated that in Ulster 1 in a 1000 people born will develop MS. Odds of 1000 to one against are astronomical when it comes to backing horses but in densely populated areas they add up to a great many people with MS.

The figures from South Africa suggest that there is a racial effect on prevalence as MS occurs in the white population, although at a low rate, whereas it appears to be almost completely absent in the black population. In the United States, however, prevalence rates for whites and blacks, although different, are much closer. There are also marked differences in prevalence between areas of similar latitude in North America and Europe, being much higher in Europe. MS is not confined to those of European stock but there certainly seems to be a relationship between high prevalence in indigenous or colonizing Europeans. Indeed, some authorities believe that

MS originated in Scandinavia some 200 years ago and spread from there across the world; an interesting idea but impossible to confirm.

There have been many detailed studies of the incidence of MS among restricted populations and particular attention has been paid to any hint that cases have formed a 'cluster'. In virtually every study of this kind groups of cases have been found, apparently unrelated by blood or marriage but clustered in some small locality. The statistical methods used in working out the odds against clusters of a relatively uncommon condition occurring by chance are complex but apparently reliable. For anyone who believes that they have found some promising clues to MS because there are six cases in a small village, it is disappointing to find how easily this could be a chance event. In those studies in which chance is statistically unlikely and some common environmental factor is looked for, nothing very convincing is found. In one survey, MS may be more common in rural areas. In another, clusters occur in certain river valleys or on sheep farms but no convincing link between these different findings can be detected. For practical purposes, within a given area there are no consistent indications that any particular occupations or habitats are unduly hazardous with regard to the development of MS. The question of possible 'epidemics' of MS is discussed in Chapter 6.

An inherited disease?

A matter of great concern to most people with MS and their families is whether the disease is inherited.

As will be seen in Chapter 6 on theories of causation, there is evidence suggesting an inbuilt, genetically determined factor that increases susceptibility to MS and the disease is somewhat more common among close relatives of those with the disease than in the general population. Large studies have shown that a child of a person with MS has a 2.5% risk of also having the disease, mother to daughter being more frequent than father to son. The risk in siblings, particularly sisters, is slightly greater, around 3%. However, MS does not behave like any of the recognized patterns of inheritable disease, such as in muscular dystrophy, haemophilia, and Huntington's chorea, for which the distinctive pattern of inheritance (recessive, dominant, or sex-linked) is known and advice based on this knowledge can usefully be given to affected families. Such advice is, of necessity, much less precise in MS and in practice is restricted to the question of possible transmission to children. The odds against this happening are, as described above, quite steep. There may be other good reasons, medical or social, for not having a family or not having a large family, but the risk of inheritance should only rarely influence the decision.

3 Early symptoms

Before describing the common modes of onset I must refer to a matter of great importance that caused me to have serious doubts on the wisdom of writing a book explaining MS to the general public. Following every surge of publicity I have been asked to see a number of people, usually young women, who are convinced that they have MS. This is because certain of the early symptoms of the disease that they may have heard described on radio or television, or read about in magazines, have a superficial resemblance to banal, everyday experiences. To lie on an arm or to sit awkwardly with legs crossed at the knee for too long causes temporary numbness, pins and needles, and even weakness, as everyone is aware. Many people do not have perfect balance between the movements of the two eyes so that, particularly when tired, vision may become blurred or double for a moment as the eyes drift apart, clearing at once on blinking or rubbing the eyes. Normally, these and other fleeting 'symptoms' are forgotten or rightly ignored as of no importance. After perhaps listening to a friend describe how MS began with numbness or double vision followed by complete recovery, it is natural to have misgivings about the commonplace events I have described, even if only in moments of anxiety or depression. Persistent fear, however, results in more persistent sensations; tingling induced by continuously breathing too rapidly, feelings of dizziness or uncertainty, and doubts about whether knocking over the milk jug was normal clumsiness or something worse. In fact, these sensations, by no means imaginary but certainly not in any way sinister, can nearly always be distinguished from the early symptoms of MS by any doctor with extensive experience of the disease, although unfortunate mistakes have been known. To brood unnecessarily and in secret is the worst possible way of coping. Fears are much more easily dispelled if dealt with promptly.

As MS can affect any part of the CNS the initial symptoms can obviously be extremely varied. The distribution of plaques is not, however, completely haphazard and there are certain sites that are particularly vulnerable. In consequence, most of the initial symptoms fall into well-defined groups.

Optic neuritis

As will be recalled, the optic nerves are part of the central, rather than the peripheral nervous system and as such, are susceptible to involvement in MS. In approximately 15% of people with MS the first symptom is known as optic or retrobulbar neuritis. These terms simply mean inflammation of the optic nerve and 'retrobulbar' indicates that this has affected the nerve in some way, behind the bulb of the eye—the eyeball. The original significance of these two labels was that in optic neuritis it is possible for the examining doctor, using an ophthalmoscope, to see the inflamed optic nerve, whereas in retrobulbar neuritis the inflammation does not reach the retina so there is nothing abnormal to be seen. Nowadays, the distinction is not regarded as important but this is what the term 'retrobulbar' means if it is encountered.

In a typical attack, the vision is noticed to be blurred in one eye. It is not always easy to tell how rapidly this comes on as, naturally enough, it is quite difficult to recognize even severe loss of vision in one eye if it does not occur suddenly. Some people only notice that there is something wrong when they accidentally rub the good eye while keeping the other one open and are then startled to find that they cannot see clearly. The eye is somewhat painful (although not red or bloodshot), particularly on looking up or to one side, and vision may continue to deteriorate for some days. The effect on eyesight varies from slight dimming of the normal vividness of colour appreciation to complete blindness in the affected eye, but the usual result is marked loss of central vision. This is most disturbing, as the act of looking at anything involves turning the eyes so that light from the object looked at falls on the area of the retina in which the light receptor cells are most densely packed. It is the axons carrying impulses from this area that most frequently lose their myelin sheaths in an attack of optic neuritis. These fibres make up a large part of the optic nerve where they lie centrally and are therefore involved in any sizeable plaque within the nerve. Fortunately, both eyes are seldom affected simultaneously.

Vision may continue to deteriorate for about a week but seldom for longer. The pain soon subsides and a week or two later, in nearly every case, vision begins to improve. The expected result is complete recovery over the succeeding weeks with eventual normal visual acuity as measured on the familiar wall chart. Sometimes, even when the lowest line can be read with ease, there may be a persistent awareness that vision is not perfect; colours may remain a little dull or contrasts of light and dark less sharp. Occasionally, central vision remains more severely affected but even here there will have been considerable improvement over the initial loss of acuity. The recovery is a characteristic example of that remarkable phenomenon in MS; the remission, a term that means substantial or complete recovery from the effects of an initial attack or subsequent relapse of the disease. Of course, many diseases remit but, unfortunately, comparatively few affecting the CNS.

There are other much less common causes of optic neuritis but an unmistakable attack is usually found to be the first sign of MS, or it may occur later in the disease. The proportion of those presenting in this way who develop other symptom and signs of MS increases with the length of follow-up, but however long this is there are always some people in whom optic neuritis remains an isolated event. This fortunate outcome is more likely if an MRI scan at the onset shows no lesions already present in the brain.

The spinal cord

Weakness

A common site from which symptoms are produced in a first attack is the spinal cord. Within the spinal cord run tracts or bundles of myelinated axons conveying nerve impulses to and from the brain and any of these may be involved in a plaque. Frequently, it is the tracts conveying impulses concerned with the brain's initiation and control of movement that are first affected. This bundle of axons is often referred to as the pyramidal tract, a name that originates from the days of purely descriptive anatomy and refers to the supposedly pyramidal shape of the tract at a certain point in its long course from the cortex of the hemisphere of the brain to the lower end of the spinal cord. Many of these axons form connections with other neurons within the spinal cord whose axons in turn enter the peripheral nervous system and eventually supply the muscles. The effect of demyelination involving the pyramidal tract is weakness, nearly always of one or both legs.

The onset may be quite rapid, particularly when influenced by fatigue. For example, the first few miles of a country walk may be accomplished normally, but weakness may make the return impossible. More usually, weakness increases over a few days or a week or two, remains unchanged for a variable period and then begins to recover. The degree of weakness in a first attack is seldom severe and often amounts to the dragging of one leg, inability to run, and some difficulty with stairs.

Sensation

The sensory tracts within the spinal cord carry impulses derived directly or indirectly from a variety of sensory receptor organs. Sensations of touch, pain, and change in temperature derived from the skin, and of pain from both the skin and internal organs are familiar enough, but there are other highly important sensory impulses that do not give rise to anything we are aware of as 'sensation' at all. We know the position of our limbs, trunk, and head in space in a most precise manner without having to think about it. Information of which we are completely unconscious is fed into the CNS from minute structures in our muscles, ligaments, and joints. This sensory input is essential for the efficient control of movement and for many of the automatic or reflex reactions of the body to changes in posture. The symptoms arising from demyelination in the sensory tracts ascending to the brain vary according to which of the different forms of sensation are affected.

A common mode of onset of MS is a sensation of numbness in the feet, ascending in a few days to the waist. Numbness implies loss of feeling, although it is often difficult to distinguish from loss of use, but it is seldom severe. A pinprick may still be felt as sharp but somehow distant. The loss of feeling may involve the bladder and rectum so that, although there is no loss of control, the normal sensation of passing water or the desire to do so is absent. Vaginal sensation may also be lost or unpleasantly distorted. There is no difficulty in walking as neither strength nor the sensory inflow from the muscles and joints is affected. Remission usually occurs after a few weeks.

These abnormal sensations are quite different from those experienced by people who have developed a fear of having MS. The latter consist of a vague tingling and numbness that moves about from one limb to another, or to the face, usually for some reason on the left side. They may be completely absent for a whole day or come on for an hour or two at any time, but are not constantly present. Such symptoms may naturally cause alarm but are not the symptoms of MS or of any serious disease.

More disabling is an initial attack in which the sense of position, the knowledge of where a limb is in space, is disturbed. When this occurs it usually affects an upper limb, resulting in a 'useless arm'. The arm is not weak in the least, but loss of sense of position and of all the essential information from the muscles and joints makes any co-ordinated movement impossible.

Bladder and bowel

The spinal cord is also involved in the reflexes that control the function of the bladder and bowel, and of sexual function in men. These are often disturbed later in the course of the disease, but also occasionally at the onset, even without any other obvious symptoms. This may present with the sudden, temporary, complete inability to pass water—acute retention of urine—usually in young women. There are other causes for this uncomfortable event and MS is certainly not the most common.

Sex

In men inability to obtain an erection is a common symptom later in the disease and may rarely be present in the initial attack, but I have never seen this as an isolated symptom of the disease. The importance of this is that men troubled by impotence who do not have any other symptoms or signs of organic nervous disease do not have MS. There are sexual difficulties for women, described in Chapter 8.

Plaques in the brainstem

Other symptoms at onset are due to plaques in what is known as the brainstem. This is the part of the brain immediately above the spinal cord through which pass all the motor and sensory tracts already described, but which is also crowded with nuclei or groups of neurons, controlling, among other important functions, the movement of the eyes and the reception of sensory information from the ears.

Double vision

The complex mechanisms by which our eyes are kept looking precisely in the same direction may be disturbed in equally complex ways later in the disease but if affected at the onset, the result is commonly double vision due to weakness or paralysis of one or more of the muscles that move the eyes. This comes on suddenly and a squint may be obvious or only detectable by careful observation. Remission is usual.

Balance and the ears

Loss of hearing is uncommon in MS, particularly at the onset, but the inner ear also contains sensory organs concerned with balance that send impulses into nuclei in the brainstem and elsewhere. If these nuclei or their connections are involved in a plaque the result may be acute disabling giddiness. There are other causes of this alarming symptom and MS is certainly not the most common. Lesser degrees of giddiness are an almost universal experience in people with no disease at all, usually the result of some passing event; an infection, getting out of a hot bath too quickly, or having too much to drink, for example. The giddiness of MS is true vertigo, that is, an extremely unpleasant and persistent feeling of rotation of the outside world or of oneself. This rarely persists for more than a few days.

Plaques in the cerebellum

Plaques often form in the cerebellum or in its connections to other sites in the CNS. This is more frequent later in the disease than at the onset. The cerebellum is a part of the brain situated at the back of the head, to which information from all the sensory systems is conveyed, analysed, and used to regulate movement. The effect of interruption of its functions is to produce loss of control of movement so that smooth action of the limbs becomes impossible and movements are said to be unco-ordinated or ataxic. At the onset of MS this may show itself as unsteadiness in walking or clumsiness in the use of one or both hands, without weakness or loss of feeling. Many normal people have shaky hands when agitated or when performing in public, but this can easily be distinguished from the effects of damage to the cerebellum just described.

Undue fatigue is common and distressing and may be the first and isolated symptom, impossible to recognize as due to MS. Tiredness is a sensation all too familiar to many people not suffering from any disease at all and, in the absence of other symptoms, should not give rise to any suspicion of MS.

These, then, are the common modes of onset in the more usual form of MS, with remissions and relapses. The list could be extended almost indefinitely as any of the multitudinous functions of the CNS could be affected, but we are not writing a textbook on neurology. All these modes of onset have features in common. In the first place there is seldom any feeling of ill health. Some authorities have tried to identify even earlier warning symptoms preceding those clearly indicating organic nervous disease and have written of 'rheumatic' symptoms or headache, in particular. I have not been able to identify anything resembling such symptoms as preceding the onset of MS. In the great majority of cases the person feels in perfect health at the time of onset and in particular there is no fever, rash, or other evidence of a generalized disease. However onset can be remarkably rapid. A young woman went to her daughter's school sports day and entered for the mothers' race feeling very fit and, as she said, intending to win. She ran about five metres and then her legs became weak and numb. She was helped up and walked with difficulty, but recovered completely in the course of the next two months. This later proved to be the first symptom of MS.

I have described the onset as affecting a single area of the CNS and this is often so. But this is *multiple sclerosis* and even at the onset there may be symptoms and signs that could not possibly result from a disease confined to a single site in the CNS. Thus, a combination of double vision with loss of feeling below the waist would clearly indicate disease in both the brainstem and the spinal cord, and thus provide evidence of multiple plaques.

Progressive MS

As mentioned in the previous chapter, in about one-fifth of people with MS, the disease is progressive from the onset. In many, symptoms begin at a relatively late age beyond the peak age of onset of the early 30s. In this group, the first symptom is nearly always weakness of one or both legs. There is nothing resembling an acute attack and unfortunately no remission either. In technical terms these individuals have 'progressive spastic paraparesis'.

Spasticity

'Progressive' is self evident; 'spastic' refers to the result of impaired conduction in the pyramidal tract (see p. 21). In addition to weakness there is loss of control of certain essential automatic reflex actions that are normally carried out through neural connections in the spinal cord. These can be tested by the doctor's rubber hammer of the comic cartoon, used to tap the tendons at the knee and ankle to stretch the muscles and induce a reflex contraction. A knee jerk is, as everyone knows, a normal finding, but when the pyramidal tracts are not functioning normally, in MS or other diseases, the knee jerk is much increased. In itself this is of little consequence, but is a sign of abnormally increased reflex activity, so that stretching the muscles in ordinary movement also causes an exaggerated reflex contraction. A result of these increased reflexes is a stiff 'spastic' leg. The toe is scraped on the ground when walking and the leg drags. Sometimes, a repetitive reflex is set up, particularly in the calf muscles, resulting in an effect best described as 'juddering'. This may first show itself when the foot is firmly pressed on the brake pedal of a car. The calf muscles are stretched and contract reflexly, causing a jerk, and this is repeated as long as pressure is maintained. The technical name for this is 'clonus'.

Malfunction of the pyramidal tract also shows itself by an abnormal reaction to firm stroking of the sole of the foot. Normally, the toes curl under, but in a spastic leg they spread out in the opposite direction. This does not give rise to any symptoms and many people find the test unpleasant, but it is a considerable help in diagnosis. It is virtually impossible to elicit this reflex on oneself and self-examination is not a good idea.

The word 'paraparesis' means weakness of both legs and is a milder form of the more familiar 'paraplegia' used when there is complete paralysis such as may follow injury to the spinal cord.

The onset of primary progression may be too gradual to allow recognition near the onset but the symptoms and signs as described above are present, alone or in combination and to varying degree, at the onset in most people with this form of MS. Other symptoms more commonly encountered later in the course of the disease are described in the next chapter.

4
The course of the disease

One of the most remarkable facts about MS is the astonishing variability in both its course and severity. Some variation is natural in chronic disease. Rheumatoid arthritis, for example, may be either mild or severe throughout its course or show great fluctuations, including complete remission. Some chronic infections, such as tuberculosis, may remain dormant for many years before eventually causing overt disease. Parallels can therefore be drawn from other diseases, but none approaches the vagaries of the natural history of MS that never cease to surprise the neurologist even after a lifetime of experience. The course of MS varies from that of an obviously grave disease to a literally imperceptible condition discovered accidentally after death from unrelated causes in old age. Most cases fall between these extremes but even so there is great variation in speed of progress, severity of symptoms, and eventual outcome.

The existence of a benign form of MS is relatively little known and certainly requires emphasis but if MS were no more than a mild nuisance there would be little point in writing a book about it. It would be futile to attempt to conceal the well-known fact that MS can be a crippling disease, capable of causing severe disability in previously healthy young people. It has been urged on me that to describe the clinical details of MS will inexcusably 'spread alarm and despondency' but I have not found this to be true. People really do not want 'the facts' to be concealed from them. With few exceptions I have found that people with MS have a strong and justified desire to know the truth, as far as it is known, and are ready to face the future bravely. Without further ado I shall therefore begin by describing the course of a severe case.

The person, most often a woman around the age of 30, has an initial attack as described in the last chapter: optic neuritis, numbness, weakness, double vision, or any of a large number of other less common symptoms, isolated or in different combinations. Recovery is usually complete within a few weeks and all is apparently well. A diagnosis cannot strictly be made after a single episode and may not even be suspected.

After an interval of perhaps a few weeks to several years new symptoms develop, usually different from those of the initial attack. Thus, optic neuritis may be followed by numbness of the legs and again recovery is complete. A further relapse, this time more severe and often including weakness of both legs occurs within the next year or two and this time recovery may not be complete—there are permanent symptoms and permanent slight disability, amounting perhaps to weakness of one leg when tired and inability to run. This pattern of successive relapses once or twice a year or once in two years continues, each time with a less complete recovery and increasing residual symptoms. Eventually, a stage is reached in which there is persisting difficulty in walking due to a combination of the spastic weakness and ataxia described in Chapter 3. The hands may also be a little tremulous and unsteady. Eyesight is usually normal. Almost certainly by now there will be symptoms of a distressing disability, failure of the normal control of the urinary bladder. A normal adult can, within wide limits, decide when and when not to pass urine. Control is exercised by the brain through connections in the spinal cord and it is these that are damaged in MS. A usual result is that reflex emptying of the bladder takes over, that is to say that when filling reaches a certain level the bladder automatically contracts. The reflexes that control the bladder are overactive so that small quantities of urine are passed frequently but fail to empty the bladder completely. The reflex activity is heightened so that the desire to pass water becomes urgent when there is only a small volume in the bladder. This urgency may lead to incontinence if there is no convenient lavatory. Less often, it becomes difficult to start to pass urine despite a strong need to do so, or the two conditions, urgency and hesitancy, may alternate.

At this stage, sexual potency in men often declines. There is no reduction in desire but ability to sustain an erection fails and intercourse becomes infrequent and unsatisfactory.

The cause of relapse

A matter of obvious practical importance is the recognition of immediate precipitating causes of relapse. Many have been proposed, among them emotional disturbance, acute infections, injuries, exposure to cold, excessive exertion, surgical operations, and pregnancy. Every neurologist will have records of striking individual examples in which one of these events has immediately preceded a relapse, but no general factor emerges and a number of supposed causes, including pregnancy and operations, have been shown not to be true. Pregnancy is discussed in Chapter 8. A particularly vexatious question is whether onset or relapse of MS can be precipitated by trauma to the central nervous system such as might be presumed to result from blows to the head or spraining the neck (and possibly disturbing the spinal cord) in whiplash injury. One school of thought even claimed that MS is caused by such trauma and sometimes succeeded in convincing a judge that this is so, resulting in large awards of damages. General expert opinion, however, increasingly rejects this possibility. There are unavoidable fallacies in trying to investigate these 'causes' in retrospect, for there is a natural tendency to remember or to exaggerate events that have an apparent relationship in time to the onset of an illness and to forget the rest. There seems to be a tendency for relapse to be preceded by some trivial infection; a cold or sore throat, but for most relapses no possible precipitating event can be identified.

Pain

For many people with MS pain is not a problem but with others it is troublesome. Backache is common and is due to the strain and excessive use put on the back muscles by walking with weak and spastic legs and by the adoption of an unwise posture. Stiff spastic limbs may ache. If spasticity is severe in later stages of the disease there may be sudden spasms in which the legs either shoot out straight or bend sharply at the knee and hip, particularly in bed at night. Usually, these are no more than annoying but the latter form, flexor spasms, are sometimes painful. The spasms are not specific to MS but may occur in any condition causing spastic weakness of the legs.

A much more troublesome type of pain that appears to be directly due to some effect of MS on the nervous system is a continuous burning sensation, usually in both legs but occasionally in other sites.

Neuralgia

Trigeminal neuralgia is an agonising pain in one side of the face that may be caused by MS but more commonly occurs in middle-aged or elderly people as a result of pressure on the trigeminal nerve by a thickened artery. This nerve,—the sensory nerve of the face—is so called because it has three branches. The pain is brought on by touching the face, eating, or talking and lasts no more than 10 or 15 seconds.

Paroxysms

These are a different kind of symptom from those that can readily be attributed to failure of conduction in demyelinated axons; weakness or loss of feeling, for example. There are a number of similar paroxysmal symptoms in MS although these are less well known than trigeminal neuralgia because they are in general much less painful. They include sudden brief episodes of unsteadiness and slurred speech or cramp-like contractions of the hand or foot. A symptom more recently recognized is paroxysmal intense itching in small areas of the skin.

A curious symptom often present at some stage of MS consists of a surge of pins and needles down the back and legs on bending the neck. You may hear it called 'Lhermitte's sign' after a famous French neurologist who described it as a symptom (not a sign) of MS. It is seldom more than a mild nuisance.

Treatment of these and other symptoms is described in Chapter 8.

The effect of temperature

Many people with MS become aware of a pronounced effect of temperature on their symptoms. A hot day, a hot bath, exertion, or even a hot drink may cause temporary weakness or blurred vision. Some people find this so unpleasant that they never have the bath water more than tepid for fear of being unable to get out. The effect may be alarming in those not used to it and causes concern about the possibility of a relapse. However, it does not last for long. One woman told me that after a hot bath she would be unable to read in bed for about three-quarters of an hour. These brief increases in symptoms are not harmful and are quite different from an acute relapse.

Any beneficial effect of cold is less obvious, partly because this may aggravate spasticity so that any improvement in strength is masked and hot weather is actually preferred. These effects of heat are readily explicable as there is experimental evidence that even a minute rise in temperature will increase the proportion of demyelinated axons that cannot conduct at all.

The effect of MS on the mind

A natural concern of anyone with MS is whether it will affect the mind. As will be described, it is undeniable that in terminal stages of the severe form of the disease there is some impairment of memory and the power of reasoning, and indeed, rigorous testing may show minor changes at an earlier stage. In most of those with MS, however, mental functions are not obviously impaired. Naturally, some are depressed but this is no more common than in the rest of the population and most remain calm and philosophical about their disabilities and prospects. This admirable stoicism is distinct from the abnormal cheerfulness or euphoria that used to be thought characteristic of MS and which is sometimes encountered in those who have become emotionally somewhat disinhibited.

Vision

Severe and permanent reduction of visual acuity is fortunately uncommon but vision may be disturbed in other ways. Most troublesome is oscillation of the eyes that causes what is seen to appear to jerk from side to side or up and down.

Later stages of MS

The stages of relapse and remission may be brief or persist for many years or even indefinitely. Eventually, however, the pattern may change and although relapses may still occur they are rare. Symptoms and actual capacity for such exertions as climbing stairs often fluctuate considerably from day to day and in the course of the day, being influenced by fatigue, temperature, morale, and no doubt other factors. Many people now experience a long period during which their symptoms and degree of disability do not change beyond these expected fluctuations. They can walk, although not easily, can drive a suitable vehicle, and can work or cope with the household and children with little more than family help. Life is a struggle but not intolerable.

Secondary progression

Eventually, if the disease is indeed in the severe form, this static period will be followed by a progressive stage: secondary progression. Walking becomes increasingly difficult. Sticks are no longer adequate support and recourse must be had to a walking frame or holding on to furniture. A wheelchair becomes necessary for outdoor excursions and eventually at home as well. Bladder control is increasingly lost with resulting incontinence but some control of bowel function is usually retained, although constipation can be uncomfortable. The hands and arms become increasingly shaky in such activities as holding a cup or spoon. This may become a serious disability quite out of proportion to any weakness of the limbs. It is known as 'intention tremor' because it becomes evident or increases whenever some voluntary action is attempted but is largely absent at rest. It was one of the symptoms that Charcot originally thought was characteristic of MS.

I have hesitated to describe the final stages of the severe form of MS, but the purpose of this book is to convey the facts of what is already universally known to be a potentially grave disease. Increasing damage to the spinal cord may lead to a bedridden and helpless state and, at this stage, mental powers are undoubtedly affected. Memory and concentration fail and it is now that the so-called euphoria, to which so much diagnostic importance was wrongly attached, may occur. This literally means a sense of well-being, which must, indeed, be rare but it is not unusual to see people cheerful and apparently indifferent to severe disabilities. With skilled nursing, whether in hospital, disabled unit, nursing home, or at home, the risks of the bedridden and incontinent state can be held at bay for many years but eventually infection may spread from the paralysed bladder to the kidneys, pneumonia may assail the lungs, or intractable pressure sores develop and in turn become infected. Weakness of the respiratory muscles makes breathing difficult. It is these complications that are the immediate cause of death.

Benign MS

At the other extreme of recognizable MS is the benign form. The symptoms at onset are entirely typical of MS but are often confined to attacks of optic neuritis and of numbness and tingling of the limbs and trunk. Remission is complete even after many relapses, and severe disability, or indeed any permanent disability at all, does not develop. I have known people who have come to regard it as quite normal that they should have one or two episodes of loss of sensation of some part of the body every year. Others may have no more than two relapses or perhaps even a single attack, typical of MS, but entirely without recurrence. Others again may have infrequent relapses at intervals of many years. In a rather less benign form some permanent symptoms, such as dragging of one leg, are present after a few years but are insufficient to interfere with work or with the enjoyment of life. Benign MS has been differently defined, most often as mild or moderate disability 15 years from the onset. In every reported series, however, a few drop out each year as disability eventually increases.

The prognosis

Everyone with MS will rightly want to know the prognosis—how things will turn out. Anyone describing the outcome of MS must acknowledge a debt to those who have had the energy and interest to follow and record the progress of their patients for 25 years or more, the most comprehensive study being conducted in Canada. Certain indications of a benign or more severe course have been established but they are based on mean or average figures and inevitably there are many exceptions. On average, therefore, women fare better than men. Good prognostic signs are early age of onset, onset with a single symptom, especially optic neuritis or altered sensation, complete recovery from the first attack, a long interval between onset and the first relapse, and several years to reach the stage of mild persistent disability. Bad prognostic signs are mostly the reverse of these but also include progression from the onset and ataxia (shaky movements and unsteadiness) from damage to the cerebellum in the first attack. These indications are necessarily imprecise and are of little use or interest to someone who has just recovered from a second relapse and needs to plan for the future.

The conclusions are in broad agreement. In 5% or less, the disease takes a particularly severe course in which death may occur within 5 years because of involvement of centres in the brainstem controlling breathing and other vital functions. The proportion of those with the benign form shows some decline with increasing duration of the disease, showing that benign MS may, after many years, eventually become progressive.

The mean time between onset and mild permanent disability has been found to be 7 years, and 15 years to reach the stage of needing help with sticks or other support on both sides to walk 100 metres. On the other hand, 15 years after the first symptom, half of all those known to have MS were walking unaided.

Survival

Survival with MS has notably increased over the years due to better care. In Denmark, where there is a national register of MS, the mean duration from onset to death was found to be 28 years in men and 33 years in women. People with MS are liable to contract other potentially fatal diseases in the same proportion as the general population, and the difference in survival between those who have MS and those who do not is relatively low at around 15%.

5
The diagnosis of multiple sclerosis

It might well be thought that any doctor familiar with the facts outlined in preceding chapters would have no difficulty in diagnosing MS correctly, but this is far from being so. In some instances, the diagnosis is certainly obvious enough but even here some caution is advisable. In series of published case histories the average interval between the first symptom and diagnosis is several years. Early symptoms, such as pins and needles, even if persistent, are often ignored or, if the doctor is consulted, are misinterpreted. No general practitioner has much opportunity to obtain extensive personal experience of the more difficult aspects of the disease. When confronted by someone complaining of tingling or numbness of strange distribution, in whom no weakness or change in the reflexes conventionally examined can be found, it is possible that the patient, usually a young woman, might be being 'hysterical'. The numbness complained of may be hard to detect by the usual methods of testing with pinpricks and cotton wool. An experienced neurologist will recognize when told that the pin feels sharp but as if there is something between the pin and the skin that this is a genuine disturbance of sensation, but it undoubtedly sounds peculiar and can lead to misunderstanding. Even if MS is considered possible there is a natural reluctance to make the diagnosis, as nobody likes to be the bearer of bad news. Apart from some special circumstances there was, until recently, no great virtue in establishing an early diagnosis but now that partially effective treatment is available it may well be decided that it is best used as soon as possible.

The diagnosis of MS can usually be made on clinical grounds, that is, by the history of characteristic symptoms and finding evidence of disease in more than one area of the central nervous system occurring at different times. There are, however, a number of diseases that do exactly this and which must be distinguished from MS. This may be difficult in the first attack and when the symptoms point to progressive damage at a single site, often the spinal cord. There is an obvious need for ways of confirming the diagnosis. Despite earlier claims to the contrary, there is no test that is 100% reliable in showing that MS, is or is not the cause of the symptoms This should not come as a surprise as this is the case for many diseases. In MS, there have been great advances towards such certainty and these are described in this chapter, but it is important to consider some of the other conditions that may be mistaken for MS. A complete list of these would be inappropriate here, and I shall not attempt it.

Diseases that mimic MS

Diseases with multiple symptoms

Diseases that can occasionally closely mimic the relapsing and remitting form of MS belong to the small print sections reserved for comparative rarities in large textbooks, rather than in a book intended for general reading, but it is interesting to consider how any diagnostic confusion could arise. These conditions, some of which (systemic lupus erythematosis, sarcoidosis, chronic Lyme disease, and Sjögren's disease) produce most of their adverse effects on the central nervous system by interfering with its blood supply. Small arteries become blocked by inflammation and thickening of their walls, and scattered regions of the CNS are damaged by lack of oxygen normally carried by the blood.

An early theory had attributed the scattered plaques of MS to the blocking of small blood vessels, in this case, veins. Although this could never be substantiated and appears to have been incorrect, it was a plausible way in which multiple damage to the nervous system might have been caused and it is certainly true that plaques are apt to form around small veins.

Surprisingly, confusion has sometimes resulted from common symptoms of the distressing but essentially harmless condition of classic migraine. In many sufferers, the headache is preceded by numbness and tingling in one arm, but this lasts for no more than 20 minutes and should not give rise to any problem in diagnosis. Young women taking the contraceptive pill are at an increased risk of a stroke with more lasting effects and this can be remarkably difficult to distinguish from a first attack of MS.

Progressive diseases

More diagnostic problems are posed by the primary progressive form of the MS. Here, there is no doubt at all that there is organic disease of the nervous system, most commonly involving mainly or exclusively the spinal cord. The problem is to avoid overlooking some quite different disease requiring different management. The most common source of confusion is with cervical spondylosis when degeneration of the joints and discs in the neck narrows the space for the spinal cord. This presents with progressive weakness and spasticity of the legs in middle age or later. It is sometimes impossible to distinguish with certainty from MS and, indeed, the two quite often occur together. The most disastrous source of error, still occasionally encountered despite modern imaging techniques, is to confuse MS of this type with compression of the spinal cord caused by a benign tumour that is often curable. As an example that I cannot resist quoting, very many years ago I was asked to see a young woman diagnosed as having MS who had been advised not to have any children. She was pregnant and naturally extremely anxious. I was able to show that she had a benign cause of spinal cord compression which was removed, curing her symptoms and allowing her to complete the pregnancy and have her much wanted baby. However, such happy endings are uncommon and in most people investigated no cause of spinal cord compression is found.

Other forms of chronic nervous disease that may be confused with progressive MS include a group of hereditary diseases which result in a variety of symptoms and signs due to degeneration in the spinal cord and cerebellum. On the whole, the outcome in these diseases is apt to be less favourable than in MS but it is important to establish the correct diagnosis because advice will be needed about the risks of transmitting an hereditary disease to succeeding generations. Inborn, congenital abnormalities of the cerebellum and upper part of the spinal cord can sometimes produce symptoms resembling those of MS for the first time in adult life and these must not be overlooked, as surgical treatment may be helpful.

The recognition of another form of spinal cord degeneration is even more important. This is the spinal cord damage that can result from deficiency of vitamin B_{12}. For practical purposes this is the result of failure to absorb the vitamin and not to a deficient diet. This causes pernicious anaemia but sometimes the nervous symptoms come first, with tingling and weakness in the legs. The patients are usually older than those with MS, but the two conditions may occasionally be confused. Deficiency of the vitamin can be confirmed by a blood test and put right by injections.

A full discussion of the differential diagnosis of MS is not appropriate here but enough has been said to illustrate the need for more positive methods of diagnosis and considerable advances have been made in this direction.

There is no specific test for MS although there have been false claims to have found one. The positive diagnosis of many diseases depends on identifying the nature of infecting bacteria or viruses or examining a portion of the affected organ or tissue under the microscope. No infective agent has so far been confirmed in MS, although many have been claimed. Occasionally, when a rare form of MS presents with symptoms greatly resembling those of a brain tumour a small fragment of brain has been removed for purpose of diagnosis but this is obviously impracticable in any other circumstances. Even when the symptoms and signs are strongly suggestive of MS it is usual and sensible to seek confirmation or exclusion of the diagnosis by means of laboratory tests.

Many of those reading this book will have undergone these tests, perhaps with little or no explanation, and may naturally wish to know more.

The cerebrospinal fluid

The central nervous system is surrounded by a clear watery fluid known as the cerebrospinal fluid (CSF). This can easily be examined without risk by means of a procedure known as lumbar puncture. Although traditionally regarded with dread, reflected perhaps by the common misnomer 'lumbar punch', when skilfully performed with a very fine needle, it is almost or completely painless, or sometimes followed by an unpleasant headache. The membranes enclosing the fluid extend further down the spine than does the spinal cord and the needle can be inserted between two of the vertebrae in the lower back without doing any harm and a specimen of CSF withdrawn and sent for analysis. In MS there is often a slight increase in the number of white blood cells (lymphocytes) present in the fluid and also an increase in the level of protein which is normally very low compared with the blood. These changes are inconstant and certainly not diagnostic of MS but the investigation is still useful, as in some diseases that might be confused with MS the changes are often much more marked.

More important is the nature of the protein in the fluid. This can be examined by electrophoresis, which is a method of displaying the different types of protein present according to their molecular weight. In about 90% of people with MS the globulin protein in the fluid can be shown by this method to contain one or several proteins not normally present. These show up as bands on the blotting paper used in the test where they have been separated by the application of an electric current, and are known as oligoclonal bands. These bands are not, unfortunately, specific for MS, but in the context of appropriate symptoms go some way towards confirming the diagnosis, whereas their absence would cause doubts.

Evoked potentials

The need to examine the CSF has been reduced by the development of a number of other methods of diagnosis, among them application of electronic techniques. It is possible to record from the scalp or the skin of the neck the minute electrical potentials induced or evoked by some form of sensory inflow to the CNS. The response to a single stimulus cannot be detected as it is swamped by background 'noise' arising from the contraction of muscles, spontaneous electrical activity in the nervous system, and other unwanted interference. If, however, the responses to several hundred stimuli are averaged they can be seen clearly while all random activity is cancelled out. This involves the recording apparatus being triggered by the stimulus so that the expected response always appears at the same point on the sweep of the recording oscilloscope. The normal response to stimulating the retina can be recorded from the back of the head near those centres in the brain concerned with vision (Figure 4a). The most constant wave in normal people is the downward deflexion that occurs about 100 milliseconds (one-tenth of a second) after the stimulus. In the figure, the responses to 250 stimuli resulting from looking fixedly with one eye at a checkerboard black and white pattern alternating once a second have been averaged. The nerve pathways between the retina and the occipital lobe of the brain are long but include the optic nerves, so often involved in MS. It all sounds complicated but is now routine, although it was exciting setting it up originally.

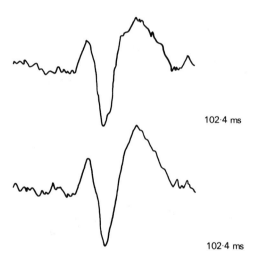

102·4 ms

102·4 ms

Figure 4(a). This shows the results of stimulating the right eye (above) and the left eye (below) in a normal person. The stimulus is a chequerboard pattern of black and white that alternates the width of one square once per second. What is recorded is the electrical wave evoked in the brain, or as much of this response as can be recorded through the skull. These electrical potentials are of very low voltage, about 10-thousandths of a volt, and what is seen here is the average of 250 responses. Measurements are taken to the prominent downward peak that is normally seen some 100 milliseconds, or one-tenth of a second, after the stimulus.

The first step was to show that during an attack of optic neuritis the main electrical potential from the affected eye, normally evoked at 100 milliseconds, was delayed and of low voltage. This was interesting but not altogether surprising, as an expected result of demyelination would be slowing of conduction in the optic nerve in just this way. What was surprising was that this delay in conduction persisted in most people after vision in the affected eye had recovered, sometimes indefinitely (Figure 4b). Here then, was a method of detecting the effects of demyelination in

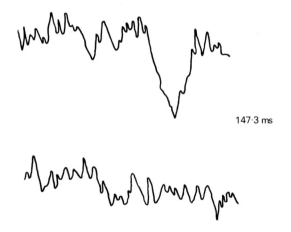

147·3 ms

Figure 4(b). This is the same test as in Figure 4(a) in a person with MS. Again, the response from the right eye is above and that from the left eye is below. In fact, no response could be recorded from the left eye as there had been a recent attack of inflammation of the optic nerve (optic neuritis) on that side and vision was poor. The response from the right eye, although of normal voltage, is much delayed at 147 milliseconds. Vision here was quite normal and had never been known to be disturbed. The test has therefore shown evidence of a silent plaque in the right optic nerve that had never caused symptoms.

the absence of relevant symptoms. It had long been suspected that plaques occurred in the optic nerve without producing a recognizable attack of neuritis and even without any symptoms at all. In people with MS the head of the optic nerve as seen through an ophthalmoscope often looks abnormally pale, whether or not there is a history of optic neuritis in the past and despite normal eyesight.

The next step was to use this visually evoked potential technique, for example, in people with progressive spinal cord disease and no other symptoms, in an attempt to show multiple lesions, that is, unsuspected symptomless sites of damage to the optic nerves, in addition to the obvious one in the spinal cord, thus affording strong support for a diagnosis of MS. Considerable success has been achieved by this method but, again, a positive result has not been obtained in more than two-thirds of people known to have MS and is sometimes positive in people who have a different disease, so, as with many things in medicine, the test is not infallible.

Other forms of nerve stimulation and appropriate recording of the response have also been used. An astonishing series of minute electrical potentials can be averaged following stimulation of the ear by a repetitive click. Electrical stimulation of a nerve in the arm evokes a recognizable response in the neck and over the scalp, related to conduction in the sensory nerve pathways through the spinal cord to the brain. Both these forms of evoked potential can be disturbed in MS, even when there are no symptoms that would lead one to suspect that such abnormalities would be found. In some hospitals, a reverse method of measuring conduction from the brain to the limbs is used. An electrical stimulus is given to the scalp and the response in the muscles of the limb are recorded so that conduction in the motor nerves can be measured. All these electric shocks sound rather alarming but none of these methods causes more than slight discomfort.

Imaging

By far the most important advance has been the development of methods for 'imaging' the substance of the brain and spinal cord.

Computerized tomography scanning

Computerized tomography (CT) scanning is a method of analysing multiple X-ray exposures so as to build up pictures of the brain as seen in 'slices'. This technique revolutionized the ease of diagnosis of many diseases of the central nervous system and spared many people from undergoing much more unpleasant investigations. It was capable of showing sites of abnormality in the brain on X-ray film in people with MS, particularly when the scan was 'enhanced' by the injection into a vein of an iodine-containing agent that accumulated in the damaged sites and was opaque to X-rays. However, even when the diagnosis of MS was regarded as certain, the scan was often normal and much more frequently when the diagnosis was doubtful.

Magnetic resonance imaging

Computerized tomography scanning in MS is now obsolete and many of the laboratory aids to diagnosis described above are used less frequently following the invention of magnetic resonance imaging

(MRI). This technique uses a powerful magnetic field instead of X-rays. The technique causes all the hydrogen atoms in the organ being examined—the brain or spinal cord or indeed any other organ—to orientate themselves in line with the magnetic field. A brief burst of radio-frequency waves is then passed through, disturbing this orientation. When the burst is switched off the spinning hydrogen atoms readjust to the magnetic field, sending off radio waves that can be recorded on film. As most of the hydrogen atoms in the brain are found in water molecules, an increased signal on MRI means that the water content of the site giving off the signal must be abnormally high and, in MS, what is seen on the films is either swelling in an acute plaque or fluid replacing normal tissues that have been lost in chronic plaques (Figure 5). The technique can be adjusted in many ways according to what it is hoped to show on the films. Apart from specialist radiologists few people, including myself, find the physics of MRI easy to understand. The apparatus is very costly to buy and maintain, but MRI has contributed greatly to the understanding of MS quite apart from the ease of diagnosis. It is a painless process, but some people find it unpleasant and difficult to lie still in a narrow box while the scanner is making alarming noises. Apart from this there are no known adverse effects.

MRI is far more sensitive than computerized tomography and shows a great many unsuspected lesions in the brain and, more recently, in the spinal cord and even in the optic nerve. Even in very early disease, when the first symptoms may be those of a single area of damage to the CNS, such as optic neuritis, multiple abnormalities may be seen when

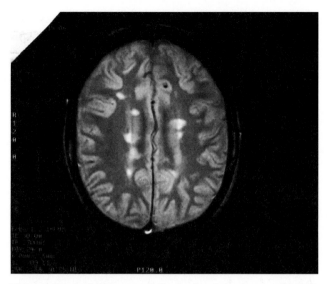

Figure 5. An MRI scan of the brain of a person with MS. The grey matter shows up normally all around the edge of this 'slice' of the brain. The white blobs near the centre are MS plaques. (Courtesy of Dr James Byrne.)

this could not have been suspected from the symptoms alone. How often and for how long plaques are present before the onset of clinical signs and symptoms is obviously difficult to investigate.

Unfortunately, none of these tests, including MRI, are genuinely specific for MS. It is possible, although unlikely, for MS to show no abnormality in any of these investigations and, conversely, for positive test results to be found in people with other diseases that clinically resemble MS. It is still necessary in those suspected of having MS for the diagnosis to be classified as possible, probable, or definite, and this is likely to continue. Certainty of diagnosis is greatly to be desired, not only because people have a right to know what is wrong with them and doctors like to know what they are trying to treat, but because understanding of the disease and its treatment must depend on accurate information.

6
Possible causes of multiple sclerosis

'The original of diseases is commonly obscure.' Dr Samuel Johnson 1777

Despite many years of intense and accelerating research, the cause of MS remains unknown. Before considering some of the many theories that have been advanced and those currently under investigation it is important to understand what is meant by 'cause' in medicine. Often, there is no problem—the influenza virus causes an attack of influenza, although why you rather than your neighbour should catch it may not be so simple. In many diseases, however, causation must be regarded as a chain that may be followed link by link, but seldom for very far. For example, a coronary thrombosis or a stroke is usually due to narrowing the arteries by fatty deposits or high blood pressure but the causes of these, where known at all, are what it is now fashionable to call multifactorial. Risk factors that increase the likelihood of hardening of the arteries (arteriosclerosis) or of suffering from its effects can be identified—heredity, advancing age, perhaps an injudicious diet, obesity, and smoking—but a single underlying reason why cholesterol should be laid down in the walls of the arteries has not been found and perhaps does not exist. We should not, therefore, be too surprised or downhearted by the present failure to identify the cause of MS. What is needed is to follow the chain of causation back to a point at which effective treatment or prevention can be applied. There are many examples where this has been done, perhaps most remarkably in diabetes. The reason why insulin is not secreted normally in this disease is even now not fully unravelled but this did not prevent the development of treatment that has entirely transformed the life of the diabetic patient. Smallpox vaccination was effective long before viruses, as now understood, had ever been heard of. Successful treatment or prevention of MS need not depend on fully elucidating the cause but perhaps the discovery of just one further link in the chain.

The quest for cause or causes of MS has certainly not failed for lack of information. Such a mass of data has accumulated that it is possible to select facts to fit virtually any theory propounded. There are, however, certain facts should be explained in any finally convincing solution. These include the unusual geographical distribution, the age range, the usual initial relapsing and remitting course, and the primary and secondary progressive forms of the disease. Individually, these can all be matched by other diseases but together they are perhaps unique.

Autoimmunity

Multiple sclerosis is considered to be a member of the large group of autoimmune diseases. The

immune system reacts to neutralize or destroy invading foreign agents such as bacteria, viruses, or trans-
planted cells. This is effected by the production of
antibodies that circulate in the blood and by cells in
the tissues that engulf the harmful invaders (and,
unfortunately, the cells of kidney and other trans-
plants, if not compatible). There are complex mechanisms that ensure that the normal tissues of the
body are actively protected from being treated in
the same way. Lymphocytes hostile to oneself are
inactivated or killed. When, for whatever reason,
this protection is faulty the body may damage or
reject its own organs or tissues, treating them as
alien. This is called autoimmunity. There are many
such diseases, some rare, but others are common,
such as rheumatoid arthritis and, like MS, follow a
relapsing and remitting or chronic progressive
course.

In MS, autoimmunity is thought to be towards a
myelin basic protein or another protein in myelin but
how this is established is, indeed, obscure. Much
might be learnt if MS occurred naturally in animals.
A disease resembling MS in many respects can be
induced in small animals by injections of extracts of
central nervous system tissue. This is known as
experimental allergic encephalitis (EAE) and is
certainly an autoimmune disease and many hopes
have been pinned on obtaining vital information on
MS by studying it. It seems, however, that EAE is the
equivalent of a human disease of the nervous system
known as acute disseminated encephalomyelitis
(translated as acute inflammation of the brain and
spinal cord) that occasionally follows infections, such
as chicken pox or measles, rather than MS. A
significant difference from MS is that animals with

EAE have been injected with myelin basic protein whereas people with MS have not. Research on EAE has not thrown as much light on MS as was hoped. In particular, it has not proved possible to assess, in the animal disease, forms of treatment intended for MS.

Much is now known of the mechanism resulting in the damage that follows the breaking of the blood–brain barrier described in Chapter 1 but the cause, the trigger that sets it off, remains unknown.

There appear to be two essential factors in the cause of MS, environmental and genetic; in other words, some external agent acting on an inborn susceptibility.

Environmental factors

Migration

The existence of an environmental factor, but not its nature, receives support from the study of the effects of migration. MS is almost certainly a rare disease in the West Indies and remains so in those who have migrated to Britain as adults. However, in their children, born in Britain and now reaching the usual age of onset of MS, the disease is as common as in the general population. Results of other migrations, particularly of white South Africans, strongly suggest that whatever the hostile factor in the environment may be, it acts in childhood, many years before any symptoms develop.

The most reliable figures are from Israel and from Hawaii, both areas of relatively low risk with good medical services and doctors familiar with MS. In both there has been an influx of migrants from areas of high MS risk—northern Europe and the United States, respectively. The results show that those who move in adult life take their high risk with them, whereas those who migrate in childhood acquire the low risk of their new home. The cut-off point was at first thought to be around the age of 15 but up-to-date results suggest that it may be much younger and perhaps only those who migrate below the age of 5 escape the high risk of their native land. Whatever figure is correct the implication is plain, something happens in early life that determines the chance of acquiring MS. This event, whatever it is, does not occur at birth or apparently in the first few years of childhood because it can be largely avoided by leaving the high-risk area within these years. Afterwards it is too late, the event, that seems to depend on environment in high-risk countries has already happened.

The external factor remains unknown but there is no lack of candidates. More rational suggestions are of excess, deficiency, or imbalance in the diet, or infection.

The effect of diet

As an example of diet there have been repeated attempts to incriminate deficiency of what are known as trace elements in the diet (elements, such as copper or zinc, that are essential to life and health but only in minute quantities). Differences in soil and geology are found but these cannot be related to areas of high or low prevalence of the disease. None of these theories has been supported by detailed investigation but this does not mean that the influence of these elements can be entirely discarded for this is a difficult field of experimentation. Out of a large number of scientific papers of variable worth, one alone seems to have remained as a kind of folk memory in the medical profession. This concerns a curious observation of a disease of myelin in lambs called, in the usual expressive veterinary way, swayback. This was plainly shown to be due to deficiency of copper in the diet of the pregnant ewes, a finding of some importance in animal husbandry. A number of those working on this project developed MS, although how analysing the soil of the sheep pasture could lead to copper deficiency or any other means of transmitting a demyelinating disease was not explained or even reasonably conjectured.

An external poison?

The possibility of an external poison is not to be lightly dismissed. There are many examples of damage to the nervous system, either peripheral or central, caused in this way. Mercury poisoning from industrial pollution was found to have caused a serious disease of the CNS in Japan, but there is no evidence that mercury amalgam dental fillings cause MS as some have feared. More extensive, but almost confined to Japan, was an epidemic of a disease now known simply as SMON from the initials of its complex (English) name. This disease, which in many respects clinically resembled MS, was found to be due to a drug widely used in Japan to regulate the bowels.

Many attempts have naturally been made to detect some toxic agent in the water or food as a cause of MS, encouraged by the remarkable geographical distribution. Lead, which is undeniably poisonous not least to the nervous system, was once a suspect but has long been acquitted. A slightly more plausible contender that will be discussed in Chapter 7 is the consumption of animal fat. Enthusiasts have maintained for many years that a high intake of animal fat is related to a high incidence of MS but the evidence is unconvincing. The original observation was that in Norway MS was less common in fishing villages where little dairy fat was eaten than in farming villages where intake was high. This now seems remote from current thinking on MS but still exerts an influence.

Infection

There is continuing interest in the possibility that the environmental factor is some form of infection. Not unnaturally, any mention of infection leads people to think of familiar infectious diseases, diseases that may be caught from contact with someone who has the disease. I must immediately make it plain that there is no evidence that MS is catching or that it can be transmitted by any form of contact. The curious pattern of MS in the relatively isolated Faeroe Isles has been cited as evidence of natural transmission of MS, even amounting to an 'epidemic'. There was an increase in new cases diagnosed between 1944 and 1960 and an attempt has been made to link this with the only notable change in environment in the islands in preceding years, the presence of British troops during the Second World War. It is difficult to believe in the transmission of a hypothetical virus from healthy soldiers to the Faeroese although this is not impossible. There is certainly nothing to suggest that MS was contracted from soldiers who actually had the disease. If MS could be transmitted by contact those at most risk would be the spouses of people with the disease. It must occasionally happen that a husband and wife both have MS but this occurs no more frequently than would be expected by chance.

Occasionally, discussion on television or radio of a possible infective cause of MS has led to people with MS being avoided for fear that their neighbours' children might catch the disease. There is no basis for this whatsoever.

It is particularly in the reporting of infective agents as the cause of MS that hope has so often been raised and equally bitterly disappointed. Many of the earlier claims were in the relative infancy of bacteriology but in at least one instance a claim, originally made in good faith, was eventually supported by fraudulent evidence. The exposure naturally had a devastating effect on the eminent supporters of the project to make a protective vaccine from the supposedly responsible micro-organism. So frequent and so circumstantial have been the claims that those experienced in the field are now apt to greet each new pronouncement with weary cynicism for they know that even the most confident claims are hardly ever confirmed by other research workers. Some of the more important recent findings must be mentioned, particularly those still under investigation. As many of these are concerned with the possibility of virus infection something must be said about these micro-organisms by way of preliminary explanation.

Infectious diseases are caused by the invasion of the body by minute forms of living organisms; mostly bacteria and viruses. Bacteria exist virtually everywhere, especially in the soil, and most of them live and multiply without ever invading man or any other living creature. Others exist harmlessly in our intestines. Those that cause disease can nearly always be identified; bacteria can be seen under an ordinary microscope, particularly when stained with appropriate dyes. They can also be grown in suitable material, usually something like soup or jelly. The presence of invading bacteria may also be inferred from the antibodies against them which are developed by their involuntary host.

There have been relatively few claims that MS might be caused by bacterial infection. However, for example, peptic ulcers, for decades attributed to worry, overwork, spicy foods, and alcohol, have quite recently been shown to be the result of a totally unsuspected infection by a bacterium lurking in the stomach from childhood.

Viral infection

Viruses are different in many ways. In the first place they are much smaller and cannot be seen under an ordinary microscope. They can be photographed using an electron microscope (EM) but this is a very different process from the intensive microscopic hunt involved when looking for bacteria. EM photographs of viruses do not at first sight suggest any form of living organism, as most viruses 'seen' in this way look more like crystals or some other inanimate object. They are, however, alive in the sense that they can reproduce themselves by simple duplication. Viruses can exist and remain infective outside the body but they can only multiply within living cells. Compared with bacteria, therefore, they are smaller, simpler forms of life and much harder to find. Difficulties in identification are such that it is only quite recently that the virus of the common complaint, German measles or rubella, has been isolated. Some viruses probably exist in the body in forms different from those seen on EM pictures. Others may persist in the nervous system indefinitely but are difficult to detect. There have been many reports of 'virus-like particles' found in tissue from MS but appearances are misleading and reports are not confirmed or are found to be irrelevant to MS.

One possibility still under investigation is that the infective agent might be a familiar virus acting in an abnormal or unusual way. A hint that this might be so is the finding that people with MS, on average, have the common childhood infections at a comparatively late age. Acute viral infections naturally stimulate the production of antibodies to the responsible virus. When the illness is over the level of antibodies in the blood rapidly falls but remains somewhat higher than before the infection. It has been tempting to attribute persisting slightly higher levels than normal to persistence of the virus. Viruses can, indeed, persist in some form in the nervous system. A common example is the virus that causes chickenpox and shingles that may lie dormant for decades. Very rarely, the measles virus can cause a fatal form of inflammation of the brain after years of normal health following an acute attack. Many, but not all, people with MS have moderately increased antibodies to a variety of common viruses, notably measles and glandular fever. After much research into these initially exciting findings the raised antibody levels are thought to be the result of a general sensitivity of the immune system in MS rather than any form of persisting infection.

Pets

Another report briefly gave rise to a different anxiety. People with MS appeared to have a lifetime of closer contact with dogs and cats than control subjects and a possible role of the distemper virus, that closely resembles that of measles, was considered. The facts are obviously difficult to obtain but larger studies have not confirmed the involvement of closer contact with animals and there is therefore no reason to banish pets from the home.

Retrovirus

In tropical countries where MS is rare, particularly in the Caribbean, a progressive disease of the nervous system, tropical spastic paraplegia, has long been known. The clinical features closely resemble those of the primary progressive form of MS but is a quite different disease, it is due to infection by a retrovirus. These viruses are difficult to detect as they may become latent or hidden in the chromosomes of the host. The AIDS virus, HIV, also belongs to this group. There have been claims, still under investigation, that a similar virus could cause MS.

Nonviral infection

When it was found that the rare disease of the brain known as Creutzfeldt–Jakob disease(CJD) was caused by an agent with unusual properties called, at that time a slow virus (now known as prions), there was much speculation as to whether a number of diseases of unknown origin, including MS, might also be caused in this way. Experiments that were claimed to confirm this were later found to be incorrect and there is no suggestion or possibility that MS is in any way related to CJD or the disease in cattle, bovine spongiform encephalopathy (BSE), that has given rise to widespread and justified alarm.

Less exotic infections have also been proposed as the cause of MS, including that common affliction, sinusitis, that accompanies every cold in the head. It was suggested that this could lead to invasion of the brain by organisms known as spirochaetes which are frequent inhabitants of the nose, but this has certainly not been proved and seems an unlikely cause of MS. A proportion of relapses of MS follow trivial infections but a direct relationship is difficult to establish.

I have mentioned only a selection of infective causes of MS that have been proposed, some initially backed by impressive evidence. None has so far been shown to be relevant and most have been long forgotten although the search continues.

Genetic factors

Since the environmental factor remains mysterious, what of the genetic influence? We have seen in Chapter 2 that incidence of MS is somewhat increased in close relatives of someone who has the disease although not following any recognizable pattern of inheritance. The risk of both identical twins having MS is much higher than in non-identical pairs, the former necessarily sharing identical genes. Possibly genes that do not carry the disease are inherited but in some way increase the likelihood of developing it when exposed to some risk factor in the environment. In MS, one such 'susceptibility gene' has been identified but plainly there are more, no doubt many more, because nothing is simple in MS.

The cause of MS remains unknown and even the initial target of the disease process remains uncertain. There is some evidence that the immediate effect of MS is on small blood vessels rather than the nervous system. The retina of the eye can be closely examined during life and, by doing so, it has been noticed that in many people with MS there is patchy leaking from the retinal veins. Examination under the microscope, when this is possible, shows that such veins are surrounded by inflammation as in an acute plaque in the central nervous system. There is no myelin in the retina so what can be seen there is not related to demyelination.

On the other hand, using very elaborate techniques only recently available, it is possible to detect subtle changes in myelin at the site of a developing plaque in the brain before the blood–brain barrier has been breached. If so, MS is restored as a primary demyelinating disease, the myelin being destroyed by autoimmunity. The responsible antibodies need not be specific for myelin but could be formed in response to some antigen, virus, or otherwise, that resembles myelin. Such 'cross-reaction' is well known in other contexts and can be highly beneficial. The eradication of smallpox by vaccination could only have been achieved because the relatively harmless cowpox and vaccinia viruses induced antibodies to the related deadly virus of smallpox.

If cross-reactivity is operative in MS, it is certainly the reverse of beneficial but the identification of the antigen responsible for triggering the reaction, if indeed such exists, would be a highly significant advance.

7
The treatment of multiple sclerosis

The treatment of multiple sclerosis is a subject that arouses intense and sometimes partisan emotions. The doctor has to reconcile the desire for effective treatment with the objectivity that is absolutely necessary to a vitally important scientific discovery, whilst not appearing to be obstructive and unwilling to try unconventional remedies. As might be expected, not all succeed in this complex task. Those with MS and their families are naturally unfamiliar with the technicalities of assessing any therapeutic agent that is not obviously an immediate cure and with the peculiar difficulties posed by the fluctuating unpredictable course of MS. Anyone with the disease will not want to wait for the results of a protracted trial before embarking on treatment for which hopeful claims have been made. Indeed, no one would wish to discourage this unless the method was harmful to health or obviously a useless waste of money, but this is not the way to discover the cure.

The efficacy of treatment

Problems with evalution

Many people find it hard to understand that there can be any difficulty in evaluating a proposed remedy for MS—just hand it out and see if everyone gets better—if only it was so simple! To establish the efficacy of any form of treatment in medicine it is necessary to compare the results in those treated by the method under investigation with those untreated or treated by other means. In other conditions this comparison may not present the slightest difficulty. For example, before the discovery of the antibiotic, streptomycin, tuberculous meningitis was invariably fatal. To save even one life was therefore a triumph. The details of the treatment were a matter for experimentation, but there was never any doubt that it worked. Only slightly less obvious was the effect of sulphonamide drugs on cerebrospinal fever, a form of acute meningitis. Here, the high death rate and the dire complications among the survivors were only too well known but some of those infected did come through unscathed. To treat a small series of patients was to be immediately and rightly convinced that sulphonamides were enormously superior to any treatment previously available. This conviction was, however, reached by comparing the results with those in a 'control' group, in this instance consisting of patients treated by other means before the introduction of sulphonamides. The difference was so striking that, again, the issue was never in doubt.

Unfortunately, the achievements of most forms of medical treatment fall far short of the dramatic, incontestable cure of previously intractable fatal disease, and consist of the partial alleviation of symptoms and the prolongation of life in chronic disease. Here, the comparison with a control group, a mere formality in the examples given above, assumes great importance and any apparent benefit in the treated group must not be described as 'striking' but in terms of significance—statistical significance. The difference between two sets of observations may be due to the influence of some discernible factor, in this instance the treatment, or to chance. Statistical methods can never totally eliminate the possibility of a chance result but can state the odds against it. Odds of 100:1 or 1000:1 are clearly more 'significant' than 5:1 or 20:1 but significance must not be confused with meaning, which depends on many factors, not least the relevance of the figures on which the calculation is based. If these are incorrect or not truly related to the outcome of the treatment, then significance becomes meaningless and misleading.

Relapsing and remitting course

The natural history of MS, described in earlier chapters, sets many traps for the unwary investigator. As an obvious example, to give the favoured remedy at the height of a relapse is to achieve what, in most diseases, would be an astonishing success as the great majority would recover or quickly improve, but no conclusion at all can be drawn as to the value of the treatment because recovery would have occurred naturally. Similarly, someone on some continuous treatment who has no relapse for five years would have reason to feel pleased but not necessarily with the treatment, as this could also be the natural course. In the assessment of any form of treatment of MS the most stringent precautions must be taken to remove the effects of chance, enthusiasm, prejudice, ignorance, incompetence, and fraud. Control results recorded previously (and perfectly acceptable in demonstrating the revolution in the treatment of meningitis), are not acceptable in MS, where the new treatment must be assessed against the course of untreated people or those treated in some other way or given an inactive placebo, observed during the same period of time in the same way and preferably at the same centre.

Random selection

At once, however, a new difficulty is encountered, that of selection. A trial in which all the severe cases were put in the untreated group would clearly be worthless, but unconscious selection by the investigator can also invalidate results. It is perfectly legitimate to exclude certain categories, perhaps those with progressive disease or with optic neuritis alone, but once the criteria are established all those who fulfil the conditions and who agree must be admitted to the trial. They must then be allocated to the treated or control group at random, that is, by some previously defined method, in which chance is the only factor involved, such as drawing a card. This is the basis of the randomized controlled trial.

Large numbers

A disadvantage of random selection soon becomes apparent in practice. Although randomization ensures that 'bad' cases are not deliberately or unconsciously allocated to the untreated control group it does not by itself guarantee that the two groups will be properly matched with regard to any factor likely to be important—age, sex, severity of disease, and a host of others. This can only be overcome by using large numbers, when the laws of chance will usually ensure that the two groups are evenly balanced in all important respects. The larger the number of patients the more likely this is to be so. The extreme variability of the course of MS is an additional reason for large numbers to be included, as results could readily be biased by an undue number of benign cases being allocated by chance to one or other group. It is possible to calculate how many patients are needed in order to detect a significant difference between the result in those treated with the agent under trial and those on a placebo.

Results

Once the trial is running, the next problem is that of assessing the results. Here, we encounter the possibility of prejudice and of the placebo effect, the well-known benefits derived from a medicine without active ingredients and given only to please the recipient. Investigators will wish to see their method of treatment proved successful or, if they are examining a treatment of which they disapprove, unsuccessful. Patients want to get better. There is a natural tendency to feel better if great interest is suddenly taken in one's previously relatively neglected condition by doctors enthusiastic about their new impressive treatment. In addition to the possible benefits, any ill effects of treatment must also be assessed. The most alarming side-effects are quite often reported by people who prove to have been taking inert dummy tablets of chalk. All this demands the most careful planning before the trial starts, but all will be wasted unless the investigation can be conducted blind. This means that neither the investigators nor the patients know whether they are receiving the new treatment. The code concealing the allocation to the different groups is broken only after a predetermined number have been treated for an adequate period, so some safeguards must be incorporated to detect a harmful effect from treatment. A fully double blind, randomized, controlled trial may sometimes be difficult or impossible to achieve. For example, cyclophosphamide caused the hair to fall out, immediately revealing who was taking it. Other methods of assessment may sometimes be unavoidable or at least acceptable but only with great reluctance.

There is no lack of people eager to enter a trial and willing to accept the chance that they might be taking dummy tablets for years. The problems of exactly what one is hoping to treat and how the results can be measured are quite another matter.

Aims of treatment

The ultimate goal of treatment is, of course, complete cure. Realistically, it is extremely unlikely that any form of treatment will be found capable of reversing all the effects of long-standing disabling MS.

Assessment

The initial aim must be for treatment that favourably influences the course of the disease. This might be achieved by reducing the frequency, duration, or severity of relapse. These criteria, particularly the number of relapses, have frequently been adopted as an indication of whether a form of treatment is being effective but there are problems to be faced. If relapses are to be counted they must be defined. When new symptoms and signs appear rapidly there is no difficulty in recognizing a relapse, but is an increase in already existing weakness or numbness also a relapse? Sometimes this is obviously so, for example, when a weak but serviceable leg rapidly becomes unable to bear weight in walking; however, such examples can shade imperceptibly into a reported (but not observed) slight increase in weakness for a few days. Is this a relapse, a natural variation, a reversible effect of fatigue due to hot weather, or merely a subjective impression not based on any real change ? It was hoped that counting and measuring the plaques seen on serial MRI scans would provide a much more accurate method of assessing the benefit or otherwise of treatment but unfortunately changes in the scans are not closely related to the rather more important matter of whether those treated feel or function any better. Further difficulties arise from the usual low rate of relapse, so that prolonged observation is needed to detect significant change.

The other immediate aim of treatment is that of arresting or reversing progressive disease: to stop people getting worse and to help them to improve. In a trial of treatment this involves standardized methods of assessing and recording the degree of disability. The results of examining the nervous system can be recorded at each visit but may be difficult to interpret in terms of significant change. A number of schemes have been proposed for recording the abnormalities in strength, co-ordination, vision, bladder control, and many other functions, and for concocting a total score or disability rating. These methods can be extremely time-consuming, which would not matter if they were always relevant and reliable, but unfortunately the scoring methods are either too sensitive, resulting in minute changes being recorded, or too coarse, so that mild but indisputable relapses hardly affect the record. All methods are susceptible to error or influence by the observer. All investigators agree that the scales used are defective but continue to use them for want of something better.

At the risk of repetition I must emphasize the rational and, I believe, eventually productive approach to the treatment of MS will be a full double blind, randomized controlled trial. This will be extremely expensive and arduous for all concerned. Even with the utmost care it is difficult to avoid pitfalls in the conduct of the most elaborate trials. The side-effects of the active agent may be so obvious as to prevent 'blinding' or the number of those treated may be insufficient to lead to a statistically significant result. It is tempting to switch the aim of the treatment away from improvement in disability to some secondary result such as changes in laboratory tests. Results of trials are often immediately criticized as inadequate in some respect. A prominent American neurologist once said 'If you want to ruin your reputation publish something good about the treatment of MS'. But things are changing.

Recent and current treatment

From time to time the International Federation of MS Societies updates a loose-leaf publication

Therapeutic Claims in MS in which many forms of treatment of recent or current interest are briefly described and discussed. Obviously, not all can be considered here and we have restricted our account to the more rational or more popular regimes.

Corticosteroids

The word 'steroid' is often used rather loosely to include the different derivatives of cortisone; corticosteroids are hormones secreted by the cortex (outer layer) of the adrenal glands (on the kidneys). The initial use of steroids or of the pituitary gland hormone (ACTH) in the treatment of MS was not based on any theory of how they might act on the disease but simply on the grounds that here was a new agent that had recently been shown to have unexpected results in a variety of hitherto intractable diseases and it was natural to try it in MS. The prolonged treatment regimes and the doses used were eventually shown not to affect the course of the disease and were largely abandoned.

However, as familiarity with steroids increased, much bolder doses were used and it is now well established that a short course of very high dosage of the steroid, methylprednisolone, either intravenously or, much more conveniently, by mouth, has a marked effect in shortening the duration of an acute relapse of MS. High doses cannot be taken for long and are given for 3–5 days. A different steroid, prednisolone, is then given by mouth in a gradually decreasing dosage for two or three weeks to avoid steroid withdrawal symptoms. A longer course increases the risk of toxic effects of steroids of which the most important in this context is osteoporosis or softening of the bones. Not every relapse needs such treatment and many neurologists would not use steroids for optic neuritis in one eye or for other symptoms, such as tingling or numbness. However, an acute attack, perhaps with considerable weakness, is frightening and rapid improvement is certainly welcome. Side-effects are seldom troublesome but undue cheerfulness induced by prednisolone may occasionally be followed by transient severe depression on withdrawal of treatment.

The beneficial effects of corticosteroids are due to their ability to reduce rapidly the inflammation present in acute plaques which is largely responsible for the new symptoms. Not surprisingly, therefore, where there is little or no inflammation, as in chronic damage to the central nervous system by MS, corticosteroids are not helpful. There has been much controversy over whether a course of steroids can affect the later development of the disease but there is no convincing evidence that this is so. Their benefit lies solely in reducing the duration of relapse, but the frequency of relapse and the degree of recovery from relapse are unchanged.

Continuous treatment with steroids should be avoided except in a small number of people with chronic MS who become dependant on steroids, getting worse each time the treatment is stopped and improving when it is started again.

Immunosuppression

The main endeavour in the treatment of MS has been towards the suppression or modification of the immune reactions of the body. The reason behind these attempts, is the theory, or fact, that autoimmunity to myelin is responsible, at least in part, for the damage to the nervous system in MS. If the body could be prevented from destroying its own myelin, relapses or progression of the disease would stop, or so the theory goes.

Many of the processes of immunity are based on the action of a type of white blood cell, the lymphocyte, that were described in the earliest stages of the formation of the MS plaque. Full immunosuppression demands the removal of as many lymphocytes as possible and there have been many trials of treatment designed to do just this.

A number of immunosuppressant drugs—cyclophosphamide, cyclosporin, and azathioprine, among others—have been used alone or in combination with steroids. Cyclophosphamide was popular in continental Europe and the United States; cyclosporin seemed to be of some help but only in severely toxic doses. Azathioprine has been extensively examined in prolonged trials. Not everyone can tolerate it as it may cause vomiting. As with any immunosuppressant drug, regular blood tests are needed to ensure that the number of white blood cells has not fallen too low. With prolonged treatment there is a small and remote increased risk of cancer. Claims of slight slowing of progression of MS have not been convincing; some neurologists prescribe azathioprine in an attempt to arrest rapid deterioration, however, it is difficult to determine whether it does any good.

All these agents are indiscriminate; they destroy all forms of lymphocytes, no doubt including many that are not involved in MS. Attempts have been made to be more selective by raising (in mice) antibodies to types of lymphocyte that are prominent in the inflammation in new plaques—monoclonal antibodies. Most of these trials have been failures. In contrast, one experimental monoclonal antibody, labelled Campath (because it was developed in Cambridge), has a marked effect, rapidly removing lymphocytes from the blood and causing a brief increase in existing signs of the disease, followed by prolonged complete cessation of activity of relapsing MS, demonstrating that immunosuppression is indeed a rational treatment, at least in the early stages. Progressive disability, it seems, is not halted.

Interferon

Interferon (IFN) is not a single substance but is a natural secretion occurring in several forms with differing properties. The name is derived from the ability to interfere with the spread of viruses. It was first used in the treatment of MS in the hope that it would interfere with a conjectured virus responsible for MS. It was given by lumbar puncture as it was thought that given by other routes it would not reach the central nervous system. Only a few people could be treated but it was considered to be of some benefit. The trial was abandoned because of shortage of interferon and the unpleasant effects of repeated lumbar puncture.

When interferon became more readily available, despite of its high cost, further trials were mounted; however, it was no longer thought that any action on an undiscovered virus was the aim. IFN-beta reduces inflammation and suppresses immunity. IFN-gamma was also tried but hastily abandoned as it was found to increase inflammation and actually aggravate MS.

Trials of IFN-beta given by intramuscular injection were shown to reduce the rate of relapse by about one-third, certainly a valuable gain although the average relapse rate is around one or two a year. However, severity of relapse, more difficult to gauge, was also reduced. Unwanted side-effects are generally tolerable, although at the beginning of a course of treatment unpleasant symptoms resembling those of the onset of influenza are common.

At the time of writing, the results of an elaborate trial has been reported. The aim was to treat MS as soon as possible after the first symptom. Of course, at that point the diagnosis is often uncertain so only people known to be at a high risk of developing undoubted MS were chosen. These can be identified by carrying out an MRI scan on any one presenting with a single characteristic symptom; optic neuritis or weakness or sensory loss due to damage to the spinal cord, or symptoms of a lesion in the cerebellum. It had previously been found that if at that stage the scan showed other lesions, not related to the symptoms, then the risk of developing MS was much increased. Even so, some of those entering the trial are likely to have had some other disease.

The presenting symptom was treated with an intensive course of steroids, as described above, and then all who agreed entered a three-year randomized, doubleblind, controlled trial of IFN-beta by injection once a week or an injection of placebo. The result was measured by the number of people who developed definite MS, usually following a relapse.

The published article naturally contains a thorough statistical analysis of the number and size of plaques seen on repeated MRI scans. These were reduced in people receiving IFN-beta compared with controls. With regard to the primary aim, that of preventing or delaying the development of clinically definite MS, the figures easiest to understand show that of those treated with placebo, 33% developed definite MS during the period of the trial whereas of those receiving IFN-beta only 24% developed definite disease. Given the large numbers treated this is obviously a statistically significant result.

IFN-beta used in this way was shown to influence favourably the course of MS in its early stages. In some ways, however, the trial was a disappointment as the conclusion was not very different from the one-third reduction of relapse found in previous trials of IFN-beta.

Attempts to influence the later course of the disease have not been encouraging. One such trial was thought to show that IFN-beta can *delay* the onset of progressive disease but this is still controversial. There is no convincing evidence that IFN-beta, given at any stage of the disease, will attain the great goal of preventing or reversing progressive MS.

Interferon is now made in the laboratory. Differing methods produce slightly different products; those used in treatment of MS being labelled IFN beta 1a and IFN beta 1b. There is no strong evidence that either form is more effective than the other. IFN-beta 1a and 1b are available under proprietary names but licensing varies in different countries.

In Britain it has not yet been decided whether interferon for MS should be prescribed on the National Health Service, and if so, in what circumstances. If eventually approved, the use of interferon will probably follow the guidelines laid down by the Association of British Neurologists (ABN). These may be summarized as follows. People who are likely to benefit from treatment with interferon are those with mild disability and a remitting/relapsing course. Those with more severe persistent disability will only benefit if they are still having relapses. There is, alas, no evidence that people with chronic progressive MS will benefit from this treatment.

Glatiramer (Copaxone: formerly Copolymer 1 or COP 1), is a synthetic product deliberately engineered to resemble myelin basic protein. When injected, this substance does not induce encephalitis in animals (EAE, Chapter 6, p. 57) and, indeed, prevents the development of this disease. A possible explanation for this protection was thought to be that the antibodies to myelin protein were all blocked by the synthetic compound locking on to them and so could not attack myelin. The obvious next step was to try the effect on MS, no doubt with some initial apprehension. After prolonged trials it was found that COP 1 was harmless, apart from some soreness at the site of injection, and reduced the rate of relapse by about one-third. There was no confirmed benefit in people with progressive disease. Glatiramer is used chiefly when interferon-beta has not proved effective, however it is not yet available on the National Health Service.

Other more or less rational treatments

Other methods of manipulating the immune system have been tried, usually with initial enthusiastic claims of partial success but later largely abandoned by all but a few optimists. These include plasma exchange whereby the blood plasma is repeatedly replaced. This treatment has been used with good results in a different autoimmune disease, myasthenia gravis, and may be of temporary benefit in some people with MS. The aim is to remove unidentified toxins from the blood.

Other methods include: total body irradiation with X-rays to destroy the immune system; removal of the thymus gland, an important source of lymphocytes; injection of antilymphocytic serum or globulin derived at first from horses but now from humans. A commonly reported result of such treatments is that one-third of those treated improve, one-third are worse, and one-third have remained the same. To an experienced student of MS this is considered to be a failure.

Hyperbaric oxygen

Hyperbaric oxygen in the treatment of MS still has its advocates although enthusiasm has considerably declined. Hyperbaric means increased pressure. Breathing oxygen at twice atmospheric pressure was found to be an effective treatment for coal gas poisoning, now no longer seen, but for little else. The original reason for trying hyperbaric oxygen for MS was that it had been found to delay or prevent the onset of EAE (see Chapter 6) in animals but many agents were already known to do this. Subsequently, the use of hyperbaric oxygen was linked to the controversial theory that MS plaques result from blockage of small blood vessels, causing local lack of oxygen.

The usual method of administering oxygen under increased pressure is for several people to be in a chamber filled with air under pressure and to breathe oxygen through a mask whilst inside. The course of treatment consisted of 90 minutes in the chamber for five days a week, these figures were used for convenience rather than for any scientific reason. The question of whether the treatment did any good ran into the usual problems: initial claims of substantial benefit were soon followed by negative results in trials in many countries. Some people have found that the treatment relieves urinary symptoms but otherwise no improvement has been confirmed and the somewhat acrimonious debate on the value of the treatment has subsided.

Diet

People with MS, as with other diseases, often ask if there is something that they can do to help themselves, rather than submitting to sometimes unpleasant and not obviously effective treatment in hospital or clinic or having no treatment at all. A number of regimes that can be followed at home without medical supervision, based on variably plausible theories of causation, have been popular, but alas have eventually been shown not to affect the course of the disease

Adhering to a gluten-free diet was not initially based on any theory but on the history, remarkable even for MS, of one person with undoubted severe MS who made an astonishing recovery while on this diet. Subsequent investigation appeared to show that in a few people with MS the gut showed effects of damage by gluten causing inability to absorb fat and other nutrients as occurs in the unrelated condition, coeliac disease. These findings were not confirmed and I hope that the diet has been abandoned in MS as it was difficult, unpleasant, useless, and even harmful.

Unsaturated fats

Another formerly controversial dietary regime, that of taking supplements of polyunsaturated fatty acids, is still followed by many people with MS and therefore merits a more detailed description of its theoretical and experimental background.

Fatty acids are a normal constituent of animal and vegetable oils and fats. The term 'unsaturated' means that some of the carbon atoms that make up the basis of the chemical formula are linked by double bonds. They are unsaturated because the structure has the potential to accommodate more atoms (the double bonds could become single bonds and link with more atoms) without breaking the essential structure of the fatty acid molecule. This is what happens when liquid fats are converted into solids in the preparation of margarine. Polyunsaturated fatty acids (PUFAs) contain several double bonds. In general, liquid natural oils contain a high proportion of PUFAs whereas fats that are solid at room temperature contain mainly saturated fatty acids.

A popular idea seems to have developed that saturated fatty acids are bad and in some way unnatural whereas unsaturated and particularly PUFAS are good and natural. This is something of a misconception as both forms of fatty acid are equally natural but occur in different proportions in different natural products, including ourselves. It is indeed likely that PUFAs are better for us and reduce the risk of stroke or heart disease; however, any link with the treatment MS is not immediately obvious.

The theory that high prevalence of MS is related to a high intake of animal fat was mentioned in

Chapter 6. The evidence for this is far from water-tight. Communities in Norway living close together but with different diets seemed to fit this pattern with a higher incidence of MS in farming villages than in those dependant on fishing. It was also thought that a diet low in animal fat was beneficial to those with MS. MS was said to be rare in concentration camps where the diet was certainly low in fats of any kind (and indeed in everything else), with increased incidence after liberation. Even these and other similar observations had been reliably confirmed they would not prove that MS is due to a diet high in animal fat or low in PUFAs but at least the idea was worth exploring.

Myelin has a high content of fat and much research was devoted to analysing the level of linoleic and other unsaturated fatty acids in the blood and in parts of the CNS affected by MS and in apparently normal areas. The findings often seemed to be important and led to interesting but eventually fruitless theories. It was suggested that people with MS might have a life-long inborn abnormality of the composition of myelin that could render it vulnerable to attack from environmental factors, such as infections, but this remained an unconfirmed hypothesis. The finding that the level of linoleic acid in the blood was reduced in MS was briefly held to be significant but was soon found to be simply the result of illness; any kind of prolonged illness. PUFAs have an effect of reducing the facility of blood clots forming in small blood vessels, a long- held but generally abandoned theory of the formation of plaques. There is more than a hint of the disappointment so familiar to those who work in MS—the failure to confirm apparently highly significant findings.

The possibility remained that, however caused, a deficiency of linoleic acid or other PUFAs might contribute to the breakdown of myelin and could be corrected by adding these fatty acids to the diet. A well-conducted double blind trial lasting two years was inconclusive. Relapses were not prevented but were slightly less severe in the treated group. Any marked benefit would certainly have been revealed.

Alternative treatments

Dismayed by the obvious failure of conventional medicine, many have turned to other forms of treatment, among them herbs, snake venom, 'rays', manipulation, and acupuncture. It is highly unlikely that any of these forms of treatment has any fundamental effect on the underlying disease process but temporary improvement in morale is frequent and worthwhile, if not bought at too high a price. For example, the Loder diet, consisting of a mixture of amino acids, was popular for a time, no doubt because it was combined with an antidepressant, but now seems to be out of favour. Procarin, delivered, at considerable expense, by a skin patch containing a variety of ingredients, has been promoted on the internet, but has not been approved in the United State for treatment of MS and has never been subjected to anything resembling a scientific trial.

The desperate need for treatment, either curative or to relieve symptoms, presents openings for fraud, by which I mean treatment offered for financial gain but known to be useless. This opportunity for enrichment has only rarely been seized and even the most apparently bizarre forms of therapy have almost certainly been fervently believed in by their proponents. This sometimes demands a remarkable talent for self-deception, a commodity seldom in short supply. Large sums should not be disbursed without seeking advice, most helpfully from the MS Society.

Finally, it is not the doctor's place to deter anyone from seeking help from, for example, faith healing or to pronounce on the possibility of a miraculous cure.

8
Coping with MS

No one who reads this chapter should think for a moment that everyone with MS must inevitably develop the more unpleasant symptoms described in this chapter. The existence of mild or 'benign' MS has been emphasized in earlier chapters. Everyone knows, however, that MS can be far from benign and it is those severely affected who are most in need of help in managing their lives.

In contrast to the search for effective treatment of the disease, the alleviation of distressing symptoms and learning how best to cope with disability are of everyday importance to people with MS and those who care for them and this chapter is devoted to these topics.

Members of the MS Society of Great Britain, when asked which symptoms caused them most distress or difficulty, surprisingly put fatigue at the top of the list (see Table).

Symptoms

Fatigue

It might be thought that the cause of fatigue in MS was the inevitable result of struggling against weak-

Symptoms causing most difficulty/distress in MS

Fatigue	65%
Bladder/bowel	50%
Balance	44%
Muscle weakness	44%
Vision	20%
Pain	18%
Muscle stiffness	17%
Muscle spasms	14%

ness and unsteadiness, and this is certainly a factor but, as described in Chapter 4, fatigue is often an early symptom apparently unrelated to the degree of disability. Why this should be so is unknown. It is certainly aggravated by hot weather and it is wise to avoid lying on the beach in the hot sun. Amantidine, a drug sometimes used in Parkinson's disease, has been claimed to be helpful but results are not impressive. Otherwise, recommended treatment involves avoiding overexertion, taking rests in such activities as housework, and readily accepting help from others.

Other causes of fatigue must not be overlooked, such as the sedative effects of drugs, including diazepam, often used to treat muscular spasms (spasticity). Fatigue is also a symptom of depression.

Depression

Being told that you have a chronic and possibly serious disease is obviously depressing news but most people with MS accept this stoically or are even in some way relieved to find that someone knows what is wrong. Clinical depression is different. It presents with early waking with persistent gloomy thoughts, hopelessness, loss of appetite, lethargy, and fatigue. These symptoms may be concealed by 'putting a brave face on it' which, although admirable, is a mistake as treatment is available and necessary, for example, in the form of an antidepressant drug. When prescribing drugs for depression, it is important that your doctor is aware of any other medication you are taking (perhaps from the hospital) because all these drugs have varying effects, particularly on the bladder, in addition to relieving depression. Amitriptyline and other drugs with a similar action can be used if there is urinary frequency with complete emptying of the bladder, but should be avoided if the bladder empties poorly as this might be made worse. A drug with a different action, such as Prozac (fluoxetine), could be used, although with caution as it can cause unsteadiness by increasing the level in the blood of carbamazepine (Tegretol) a drug sometimes used to control pain. Whether depression is an actual symptom of MS, caused by damage to some part of the central nervous system, is doubtful.

Bladder and bowel problems

The correct management of bladder symptoms is of great importance. The first symptoms usually occur when there is a relatively slight difficulty in walking and consist of increased frequency of passing water and an urgent need to do so. This is inconvenient and may result in embarrassing incontinence, but it is not serious. If the bladder is being completely emptied, the frequency and urgency can be helped by drugs, such as oxybutynin or tolterodine, the latter being less likely to cause a dry mouth. Desmopressin nasal spray greatly reduces frequency and is particularly useful when used at night as frequently getting out of bed to pass water, perhaps with weak legs, is exhausting. The spray should not be used more than once in 24 hours and should not be given to the elderly or anyone subject to seizures. The fluid intake should not be restricted. Drinking cranberry juice makes the urine acidic and germs do not like this, thus reducing the chance of infection.

As time passes, despite urinary frequency, the bladder may not be emptied completely although this often comes as a surprise when a simple scan shows a large unsuspected volume of residual urine. The stagnant urine increases the risk of infection and of stones in the bladder. If possible, therefore, the bladder should be drained once a day. This can be achieved by passing a catheter into the bladder through the urethra, the natural passage. Many people learn how to do this for themselves, after instruction by a nurse. Low friction catheters, lubricated with water, are easy to use. Of course, some degree of manual dexterity is necessary but it is remarkable how well people manage. The bladder can also be stimulated to empty by applying a vibrator (a Queen Square stimulator) to the lower abdomen. This is also useful when there is difficulty in starting to pass urine. Emptying the bladder naturally reduces the volume of any incontinence but does not prevent it. For men there is a reasonably effective urinal with a device like a condom placed over the penis but a satisfactory urinal for women has yet to be invented. Kykie bed protectors are very absorbent.

Eventually, frequent incontinence may require that the catheter be left in. This increases the risk of urinary infection but reduces damage to the skin from being soaked in urine. Problems are frequent. Urine may leak round the catheter; the catheter may block; spasm of the adductor muscles may hold the legs together so that attending to the catheter is impeded or impossible. The spasm may be overcome by injections of botulinum toxin into the adductor muscles, given by your local consultant in rehabilitation medicine. A blocked catheter can be washed out by a nurse and, if blocking is recurrent, the bladder can be cleared of stones and sludge by a urologist using a cystoscope, but this may require a general anaesthetic. Sometimes stones can be broken up using a high speed vibrating device, a procedure not needing an anaesthetic. It is often safer and more convenient to use a suprapubic catheter, inserted through the lower abdomen by a small operation.

Constipation is common but only rarely extreme, causing severe distension. Laxatives should be used with caution as they can cause incontinence and a glycerine suppository or Microlax enema used regularly are often effective. Another laxative, Movicol, retains fluid in the bowel and has proved useful. Simple measures, such as linseed grains on the breakfast cereal, a good fluid intake, and fresh fruit in the diet should not be neglected. In extreme cases, manual removal of faeces by a nurse may be necessary.

Persistent and disabling incontinence may be tackled by a new technique known as ACE (anterior colonic enema) whereby the appendix is a brought to the skin surface and the bowel is flushed with water through the appendix.

Sex

Many people with MS, and indeed with many other diseases, are too shy to mention problems with sexual intercourse. Doctors should know this and should specifically ask about it but doctors are sometimes shy too. Do not be afraid to speak up, however embarrassing this may be, as help is often possible. Failure of erection is common as a symptom of MS but other causes should be considered, particularly drugs such as baclofen, used to treat spasticity. Sildenafil (Viagra) is often successful in restoring potency. Mechanical devices causing erection by restricting the base of the penis may also be helpful. Other methods involving injections into the penis or inserting medicaments into the urethra, the natural passage of the penis, are taught in clinics specializing in this problem.

Women also have difficulties with intercourse. Adductor spasm of the thighs can be treated with botulinum toxin injections. If an indwelling catheter is needed an active sex life requires that this should be suprapubic. Loss of vaginal secretions requires a water-soluble lubricating jelly, not Vaseline. Unfortunately, blunting of sensation is more difficult to help but SPOD (see Appendix) can tell you where to buy a mains-generated oscillator that can help.

Balance

Loss of balance, often combined with loss of strength, requires some form of support—a stick or a suitable walking frame. It should be possible to try out different types of frame under the supervision of a physiotherapist to find which is most suitable.

Tremor

Tremor of the arms, sometimes also involving the head, varies from a mild nuisance to severe disability, prohibiting any useful movement of the upper limbs. Although many drugs have been tried they are only rarely helpful, propranolol in quite large doses is most likely to be effective. It cannot be taken by anyone liable to asthma. Some have claimed benefit from cannabis. Surgery to destroy particular small areas of the brain can greatly reduce tremor, although much less reliably than in Parkinson's disease. The aim is to provide one useful arm. A slightly different approach is to insert a stimulator in the same area of the brain but this needs frequent adjustment and long journeys to the few centres offering this technique.

Environmental control systems are available after assessment by a consultant in rehabilitation. These ingenious machines, known as Possum or Steeper according to make, allow someone with poor hand function, using a squeeze switch (Figure 6), to open the door, work a computer, use a telephone or switch on lights or television, or even work a page turner (Figure 7). Chin switching can be used by those with no hand function.

Weakness

Some weakness of the lower limbs is almost invariable in established MS. Certain patterns of weakness can be recognized, particularly difficulty in lifting the foot when walking. Splints are awkward to manage but an ingenious device, named the Odstock drop foot stimulator (after the centre where it was developed) is sometimes helpful particularly if the weakness is mainly on one side. As shown in Figure 8, on contact with the ground, an electrode on the heel sends a current that stimulates the muscle that lifts the foot.

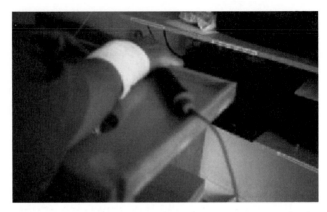

Figure 6. Grasp or squeeze switch which is useful for severe tremor.

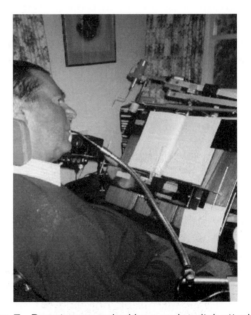

Figure 7. Page turner worked by a suck switch attached to an environmental control system–an electronic device used to control electrical equipment such as door openers, telephone, TV, and hi-fi.

The fear is often expressed that using a wheelchair to make life easier will accelerate deterioration
in walking. There is no evidence for this, indeed,
the energy saved will make walking and standing
easier. If a wheelchair is needed a wheelchair thera-
pist should be consulted to ensure that the chair
provides essential support and does not aggravate
the pain and discomfort of spasticity. The ideal
posture is shown in Figure 9 with the thighs at a
right angle to the trunk, the knees also flexed to a
right angle, and the feet on footplates. The tendency to slip forward, which worsens spasticity, can
be prevented by a ramped cushion, as shown.
Prolonged sitting causes swollen legs, which every-
body dislikes, some to the extent of keeping the feet
up. Swelling can be relieved by appropriate stock-
ings and specialized massage (address in Appendix
for the address of the British Lymphology Society),
not available everywhere.

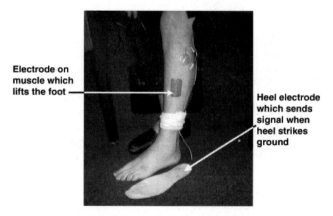

Electrode on
muscle which
lifts the foot ——

Heel electrode
which sends
signal when
heel strikes
ground

Figure 8. Functional electrical stimulator for foot drop.

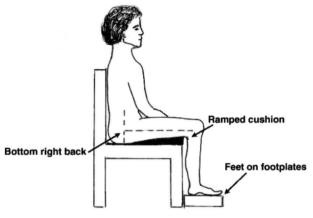

Figure 9. The ideal posture if there is spasticity of muscles.

Vision

Complaints of failing vision are common although often nothing to do with MS and can be put right with reading glasses. There is unfortunately no reliable treatment for the disorders of eye movement that cause what is looked at to jerk from side to side or up and down. Very skilled use of botulinum toxin is occasionally successful.

Pain

Trigeminal neuralgia (Chapter 4) nearly always responds to carbamazepine (Tegretol). Much more difficult to treat is burning pain in the legs. Carbamazepine may be helpful and also the antidepressant, amitriptyline. Gabapentin, a drug introduced to treat epilepsy, has been found to reduce both pain and spasticity but is apt to cause unwelcome weight gain. Nabilone, an extract of cannabis, is not licensed for use in MS and is extremely expensive, but in brief trials has been helpful. It should not be prescribed for people with impaired memory. A trial of cannabis itself is in progress.

Spasticity

As explained in Chapter 3, spasticity is the result of increased reflex activity induced by stretching the muscles and tendons, most importantly in the legs. It is common in MS because of damage to the descending motor pathways in the spinal cord that normally control these reflexes. In walking, the effect of spasticity is to hold the legs straight at the knees with the feet pointing downwards, resulting in a stiff and awkward gait and scraping of the toes on the ground. An advantage of the legs being held in this position is that they form efficient props, allowing the upright position to be maintained. Spasticity of this degree in legs already weakened is uncomfortable but sometimes assists walking rather than impeding it. To abolish spasticity in this instance may result in weak legs that can no longer support the body's weight. Theoretically, it should be possible to reduce the overactivity of the stretch reflexes without producing weakness and a number of drugs have been claimed to do just this, but none of them has been found to make it easier to walk.

However, there are other reasons for reducing spasticity. The legs are often cramped and painful, especially in bed at night. The most effective drug is baclofen, best given at night initially, the dose being carefully increased to relieve pain without excessive weakness that would, for example, make it difficult to get out of bed to pass water. Another drug,

Dantrium is also effective. Tizanidine is preferable if the legs are already very weak and there is a risk of falling, as its action is milder. Diazepam is also active against spasticity but is soporific which sometimes may be an advantage.

Another feature of spasticity is spasm in the legs. Sometimes the legs shoot out straight, which is very awkward for someone in a wheelchair but in more advanced disease the legs suddenly bend at the hips and knees. These flexor spasms are often painful and distressing and respond less well to baclofen. Spasms may be aggravated by anything that acts as a stimulus to the stretch reflexes: a blocked catheter, urinary infection, pressure sores, an ingrowing toenail, or emotional stress. Standing frames are beneficial in reducing spasticity and allowing some exercise as an aid against osteoporosis (brittle bones) but are elaborate and need help from a expert physiotherapist such as may be found at an MS centre.

As mentioned above, botulinum toxin is particularly useful in treating spasticity in the muscles that bring the thighs together. It is given by injection into the muscles and acts by blocking the chemical that is normally released from nerve endings and causes muscular contraction. This treatment is given by rehabilitation consultants and some neurologists. The effect lasts about three months.

In very severe and intractable spasticity, baclofen can be given by an electronic pump into the cerebrospinal fluid around the spinal cord. This is not without complications and is usually reserved for people with spinal cord injury rather than MS. Pump refills can involve long journeys to specialist centres.

Other considerations

Difficulty in swallowing

This is relatively uncommon but is an important symptom as it can lead to repeated chest infections from inhaling food or fluid. Reduced food intake causes malnutrition, impaired healing of pressure sores, and decreased resistance to infection. Inadequate fluid intake increases the risk of urinary infection.

Thickened drinks or yoghurt are less liable to slip down the wrong way. If such means are unsuccessful nutrition can be maintained by a percutaneous endoscopic gastrostomy (PEG). This consists of a small tube leading from the stomach to a hole in the abdominal wall, held in place by a small balloon. Artificial liquid foods can be given this way; and although it still possible to eat in the normal way, there is the continued risk of inhaling food. When the PEG is replaced after a few months the tract into the stomach will have become well established and a more cosmetically acceptable PEG, lying flush with the skin, can be used.

Osteoporosis

Thinning of the bones, with risk of fracture, occurs particularly in women past the menopause, although men are also affected. Osteoporosis can be detected by a bone scan that can be arranged by the family doctor. The risk is increased by lack of exercise, by steroid treatment, by smoking and excessive alcohol. Effective treatment is now available. Vitamin D and calcium supplements may be sufficient. In women, those most at risk, hormone replacement therapy (HRT) will protect the bones and for those who cannot take this there are drugs called biphosphonates which are indicated if a scan shows definite osteoporosis.

Pressure sores

Anyone, from whatever cause, lying or sitting immobile for a long period is at risk of developing pressure sores. This is because it is normal to shift our position frequently without thinking about it, allowing flow through small blood vessels compressed by the weight of the body against a firm surface. When weakness, particularly of the arms, makes this impossible the continued pressure deprives the skin of blood and oxygen so that it may die. And not only the skin; pressure sores may extend through the muscle right down to bone. Such sores are a particular threat to people with MS as loss of sensation may prevent any warning of trouble and incontinence may further damage the skin. The utmost care must be taken to prevent pressure sores as they are not easy to heal.

Particularly when the bottom is numb, the area should be inspected daily, using mirrors if there is no carer. The temperature of bath water should be checked with a thermometer. A pressure-relieving cushion should be used in a chair. Many people using a wheelchair are able to transfer themselves unaided between wheelchair and bed, a most useful achievement. Using both an air cushion and an air mattress may make this difficult or impossible so that a relatively firmer gel cushion and foam mattress should be used. A tilt-in-space chair also helps to relieve pressure. A particular time of risk is when admitted to hospital for some unrelated condition. The medical and nursing staff may well be unfamiliar with MS and the need to protect the skin by using an air mattress may not always be understood or an appropriate mattress may not be available at short notice.

Treatment of an established sore requires several weeks in bed on an air mattress with frequent changes of posture. Many different dressings have been claimed to be helpful. Some hydrogel dressings can fill the cavity and assist in removing dead tissue. Foam dressings, such as Allevyn, do not adhere to the wound and do not cause injury each time the dressing is changed

Nutrition must be preserved with a high protein diet and essential vitamins. Sometimes plastic surgery may be needed but is not always successful.

Pregnancy

For many years it was firmly held that pregnancy and childbirth were absolutely forbidden in MS as it was thought to be highly dangerous. This has repeatedly been shown to be untrue. During the nine months of pregnancy the relapse rate is, on average, somewhat reduced. In the three months following delivery the risk of relapse, again on average, is slightly increased, so that the total effect is neutral. Epidural anaesthesia in labour is safe and there is no risk in breast-feeding. A large family is usually inadvisable, but there are exceptions, including a woman who proudly brought up no less than seven children.

Surgery

It used to be considered (without any evidence) that operations and anaesthetics were dangerous in MS and were apt to bring on relapse. However, it has been shown repeatedly that most operations are not followed by any setback and necessary surgery should certainly be accepted without any such fears. On the quite unscientific idea of 'not rocking the boat' purely cosmetic operations are best avoided. Dental extractions can safely be carried out under local anaesthesia.

Inoculations

Inoculations against infections, including influenza, have been shown not to cause relapse of MS.

Financial support

Welfare benefits vary from country to country. In the UK, the Disability Living Allowance (DLA) is not means tested and can provide money for personal care with a mobility component for those who are virtually unable to walk. It must be applied for before the 65th birthday. After that age, Attendance Allowance can be applied for if help is needed with personal care but there is no mobility component. Those who have received the mobility component of the DLA will continue to receive this after the age of 65. It is essential to remember this when people with MS are approaching this age. Advice can be obtained from Citizens' Advice Bureaux and Disability Income Group (see Appendix). People on income support do not pay for prescriptions. Someone with MS, if not receiving income support, can apply for free prescriptions if they are unable to leave the house without the help of another person.

Work

Keep as active as you can, short of undue fatigue. Many employers will do their utmost to find appropriate work, but it is often getting to work that is the problem. There are 'Access to Work' schemes providing funds to assist with this problem. Explore the possibilities of a modified car with hand controls. It is extremely important to maintain contact with people who are not disabled and not to accept isolation from the accustomed social round.

Physiotherapy

People with MS are often disappointed when they are discharged from the physiotherapy department. The benefit from physiotherapy must be balanced against fatigue and weakness that may result from too much exertion and particularly from long, exhausting journeys to the clinic. On the other hand, a regular aerobics exercise programme can reduce depression and improve social interaction. The carer can be taught to do passive stretches to reduce stiffness and help to prevent contractures. However, research in other conditions suggests that rehabilitation is more effective if carried out by a multidisciplinary team.

Multidisciplinary teams involve therapists seeing patients independently of other members of the team and often in individual departments. An even better arrangement is the interdisciplinary team in which members work together, often from the same office, sharing expertise, notes, and training. The aim is for those from different disciplines, occupational therapy, physiotherapy, speech therapy, and nurses trained in rehabilitation to have joint sessions with the person with MS and have regular team meetings. Relearning how to transfer from bed to chair when the skin has become vulnerable to pressure sores can be a key issue in maintaining independence and sometimes there must be a compromise between safety of the skin and ability to transfer. The goal of transferring in the most effective way involves physiotherapy, occupational therapy, and the rehabilitation nurse working with the patient in a co-ordinated programme. If transfers are really precarious, 'through floor' lifts are safer than stair lifts and increase independence. Social Services employ their own occupational therapists to advise on adaptations (Figures 10 and 11). Assessment in hospital of people with MS and significant disability by such a team at the National

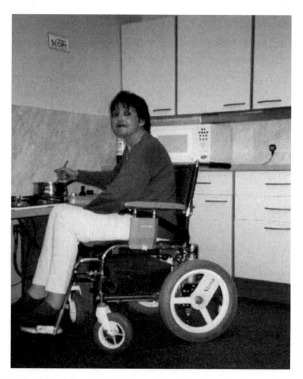

Figure 10. Adapted kitchen with wheelchair height cooking surfaces.

Hospital for Neurology and Neurosurgery has shown that disability and quality of life can be improved even if the neurological defect cannot.

The MS Society of Great Britain and Northern Ireland, in collaboration with the National Hospital and with much input from people with MS and their families, have drawn up guidelines for service provision for those with MS. In the early stage of the disease the need for a clear and certain diagnosis is emphasized. Support and counselling and access to information are key areas. People with moderate or severe disability should have access to a multidisciplinary team and adequate respite care. There

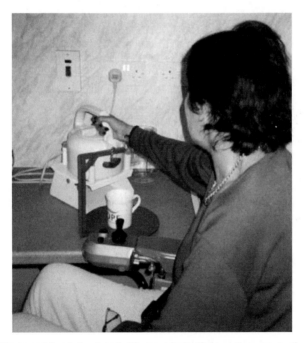

Figure 11. A tipping kettle can help if there is arm weakness or tremor.

should be appropriate facilities for long-term care and for care in the community.

Sadly, provision falls far short of this. Only 8% of members of the British MS Society who have the disease had been referred to a consultant in rehabilitation medicine. Too few consultants in the specialty have been appointed and skills in rehabilitation have been much underused. People with MS need much more than routine visits to a crowded neurological clinic.

The Multiple Sclerosis Society

This is a worldwide charitable society with local branches. Half the money it raises is devoted to supporting research and half to care of people with MS. In some areas, there are welfare officers and MS nurses to give practical advice and help. Some people do not like attending Society meetings because they are distressed by seeing people with more severe disease. Apart from this, meetings serve a useful purpose as local information on such matters as respite care can be exchanged and tips on coping passed on to people with MS, their carers, and doctors. It is helpful to share these experiences and problems.

The internet is a useful means of communication if you have access to a computer and the MS societies have web sites (see Appendix).

The future

In successive editions of this book hope has been expressed that the increasing volume of high quality research will lead to the discovery of the cause and cure of MS. This has not yet been achieved but it is encouraging that methods of reducing the frequency of relapse are now available and work is in progress to determine the best way to use interferon. The progressive form of the disease, either primary from the onset or secondary after a remitting and relapsing stage, has not yet been reliably shown to be influenced by manipulation of the immune system, probably because some different form of damage to the nervous system is involved by which the axons are increasingly stripped of myelin and eventually lost.

Methods of reforming myelin, at least in the most important areas of the brain or spinal cord, are being considered but there are many risks and difficulties in surgically introducing oligodendroglial cells that could form myelin and that would be able to move to where they were most needed. Perhaps primitive stem cells, that can be transformed into a number of types of specialized cells, may eventually be used to repair the nervous system. That such treatment can even be discussed is evidence of adventurous thinking on the still baffling problems of multiple sclerosis.

Partial or complete recovery from severe weakness or even paralysis is a remarkable feature of relapsing and remitting MS. Explanations have included relief of inflammation and swelling in plaques that have caused the symptoms and, less certainly, remyelination of the affected axons. A very recent suggestion, supported by interesting evidence, is that recovery may be due to other parts of the brain taking over the functions of the axons that have been put out of action. Such 'plasticity' of the brain is a well-established phenomenon and there are methods of encouraging it that might conceivably be applied to MS.

On a more immediately attainable level the combined resources of the general practitioner, neurologist, rehabilitation physician, and the multi-disciplinary team will help people with MS feel that they have the support that they need to manage their disease.

Appendix

MS Society addresses

Australia
34 Jackson St
Toorak
Victoria
3442
Tel: (61) 3 9828 7222;
Fax: (61) 3 9826 9054
Email: public@mssociety.com.au

Canada
Suite 1000
250 Bloor St East
Toronto
Ontario
M4W 3P9
Tel: (1) 416 922 6065;
Fax: (1) 416 922 7538
Email: info@mssoc.ca
http//www.mssociety.ca

Great Britain and Northern Ireland
372 Edgware Road
London
NW2 6ND
Tel: 0208 438 0700;
Fax: 0208 438 0701
Helpline: 0808 800 8000
(9am-9pm Mon-Fri)
Email: info@mssociety.org.uk
http//www.mssociety.org.uk
34 Annadale Avenue
Belfast
BT7 3JJ
Tel: 01232 802 802
Fax: 0123 802 803
Email: info@mssociety.org.uk

Rural Centre
Ingliston
Edinburgh
EH28 8N2
Tel: 0131 472 4106
Fax: 0131 472 4099

New Zealand
PO Box 2627
Wellington 6005
Tel: (64) 4 499 4677;
Fax: (64) 4 499 4675
Email: tjordane@mssocietynz.co.nz

Republic of Ireland
MS Society of Ireland
Royal Hospital Donnybrook
Bloomfield Ave
Morehampton Rd
Dublin 4
Ireland
Tel: (353) 1 269 4599;
Fax: (353) 1 269 3746
Email: info@ms-society-ie
http//www.ms-society.ie

Republic of South Africa
South Africa National MS Society
295, Villiers Rd
Walmer
Port Elizabeth 6070
Tel: (27) 41 581 2900;
Fax: (27) 581 5705
Email: sanmss@jhb.lia.net

United States
National MS Society
773 Third Avenue
New York
NY 10017
Tel: (1)212 986 7081 3240;
Fax: (1) 212 986 7981
Email: info@nmss.org
http.//www.nmss.org
Toll Free No 1–800-FIGHT MS

Zimbabwe
MS Society of Zimbabwe
PO Box BE 1234
Belvedere
Harare
Zimbabwe
Tel: (263) 4 740 472; Fax: (263) 4 740 472 (ask for a line)
Cell (263)11204478
Email: therobs@turtle.icon.co.zw

Other useful addresses

British Lymphology Society
Administration Centre
PO Box 1059
Caterham
Surrey
CR3 6ZU
Tel: 01883 330253; Fax: 01883 330254
Email:
helensnoad@blsac.demon.co.uk

Crossroads Care (a sitting service, while carers go out)
10 Regent Place
Rugby
Warks CV21 2PN
Tel: 01788 573653

DIG (Disability Income Group)
PO Box 5743
Finchingfield
Essex
CM7 4PW
Tel: 01371 1621

Disabled Living Foundation
380–384 Harrow Rd
London
W9 2HU
Tel: 0207 2896111;
Fax: 0207 2662922;
Helpline: 0845 130 9177
www.dlf.org.uk

Disabled Living Centres Council
Redbank House
4 St Chads
Manchester
M8 8QA
Tel: 0161 834044; Fax: 0161 835 3591
www.dlcc.demon.co.uk

National Association of Citizens' Advice Bureaux
Middleton House
115–123 Pentonville Rd
London
N1 9LZ
Tel: 0207 833 2181
http:www.nacab.org.uk

REMAPS (a group of engineers who try to devise solutions to difficult problems)
Hazeldene
Ightam
Sevenoaks
Kent
TN15 9AD
Tel: 01723 883818

SPOD (Sexual and Personal Relationships of the Disabled)
286 Camden Road
London
N7 0BJ
Tel: 0207 6078851

INDEX

Index

Index